QUESTIONS
· ABOUT THE ·
BEGINNING
OF LIFE

QUESTIONS ABOUT THE BEGINNING OF LIFE

Christian Appraisals
of Seven Bioethical Issues

EDITED BY

Edward D. Schneider

AUGSBURG Publishing House • Minneapolis

QUESTIONS ABOUT THE BEGINNING OF LIFE
Christian Appraisals of Seven Bioethical Issues

Copyright © 1985 Augsburg Publishing House

Scripture quotations unless otherwise noted are from the Revised Standard Version of the Bible, copyright 1946, 1952, and 1971 by the Division of Christian Education of the National Council of Churches.

Library of Congress Cataloging-in-Publication Data

QUESTIONS ABOUT THE BEGINNING OF LIFE

Bibliography: p.
1. Human reproduction—Moral and ethical aspects.
2. Genetic counseling—Moral and ethical aspects.
3. Fetus—Diseases—Diagnosis—Moral and ethical aspects.   4. Infants (Newborn)—Diseases—Treatment —Moral and ethical aspects.   I. Schneider, Edward D., 1936–
QP251.Q45   1985   241'.66   85-15617
ISBN 0-8066-2167-2

Manufactured in the U.S.A.   APH 10-5360

1   2   3   4   5   6   7   8   9   0   1   2   3   4   5   6   7   8   9

860054€8

Contents

Contributors

Edward D. Schneider, Assistant to the Presiding Bishop, The American Lutheran Church, Minneapolis, Minnesota

Paul T. Jersild, Dean of Academic Affairs and Professor of Theology and Ethics, Lutheran Theological Southern Seminary, Columbia, South Carolina

Janet Dickey McDowell, Adjunct Professor of Religion, Roanoke College, Salem, Virginia

James H. Burtness, Professor of Systematic Theology, Luther Northwestern Theological Seminary, St. Paul, Minnesota

James M. Childs Jr., Academic Dean and Associate Professor of Christian Ethics, Trinity Theological Seminary, Columbus, Ohio

Edmund N. Santurri, Instructor in Religion, St. Olaf College, Northfield, Minnesota

Hans O. Tiefel, Professor of Religion, College of William and Mary in Virginia, Williamsburg, Virginia

Preface

Our society is the most technologically advanced society in human history. Nowhere is this more apparent than in the array of medical technology available to us. We have celebrated these medical triumphs, and we press on for more.

At the same time we have come to recognize that technology of any sort is not an unqualified good. New discoveries and new technologies bring possibilities of new evil as well as good, new suffering as well as relief. The same medical gadgetry that can preserve and extend life, for example, can also prolong suffering and the process of dying.

Because of the ambivalent character of modern medical technology, we are confronted with complex questions and decisions not dreamed of by our predecessors. This book examines seven such questions that focus on the beginning of life. Some of these questions relate to very personal decisions. Questions pertaining to artificial insemination or *in vitro* fertilization, for example, are intensely personal, even though they obviously involve legal and social-policy issues. Other questions, such as some of those posed by genetic manipulation, are more immediately directed to social-policy issues.

Because these are questions pertaining to life-and-death is-sues, the church has a concern to be involved. In confronting such questions, persons of faith search their own religious tra-ditions looking for assistance or guideposts when they make decisions. For this reason, The American Lutheran Church through its Office of Church in Society, and the Lutheran Church in America, through its Department of Church in So-ciety, joined in a cooperative effort to provide resources in this area. Staff coordinators of the overall project were Paul Nelson and myself, both of us then serving in the Church in Society units of our respective churches. We were assisted by an ad-visory committee of three persons: Chaplain William Adix, Dr. Joan Bennett, and Dr. Chris Brelje.

It has been my pleasant task to coordinate the development of this book. As editor I wish to express my appreciation to members of the advisory committee and others for their reading of the manuscripts and their helpful suggestions.

Finally, I wish to thank each of the contributors to this volume for their part in helping us all to wrestle more earnestly and thoughtfully—in light of our faith commitments—with questions about the beginning of life.

EDWARD D. SCHNEIDER

1

Artificial Insemination

—————Edward D. Schneider—————

In our society most young people still marry with the expectation that they will have children. Fertility is almost universally assumed on the part of such people, but it is estimated that 10–15% of such marriages prove to be barren. In approximately 40% of those cases, barrenness is the consequence of male infertility.[1]

When couples find themselves childless because of male infertility, they have several choices. They can remain childless and learn to cope with their disappointment, or they can adopt someone else's child. With declining numbers of infants available for adoption and frequent delays in the adoption process, however, adoption is becoming less of an option for many people. A third alternative is artificial insemination.

Artificial insemination is a relatively simple medical procedure by which semen obtained by masturbation is deposited by means of a syringe in or near the cervix of the woman's uterus. Artificial insemination is of two basic types: *homologous insemination*, or artificial insemination by husband

(A.I.H.), when the semen is obtained from the husband; and *heterologous insemination*, or artificial insemination by donor (A.I.D.), when the semen is obtained from a donor. A.I.H. is used occasionally when for physical or psychological reasons insemination through intercourse is problematic, or in the case of oligospermia (deficient sperm count) when sperm from several ejaculates are pooled for use in a single insemination. Since A.I.H. presents few legal, social, or ethical problems, this chapter will focus primarily on A.I.D.

Artificial insemination by donor (A.I.D.) is "medically indicated" in cases of complete or virtually complete male infertility, or in cases in which the husband fears transmitting genetic disease. A.I.D. is also utilized to provide natural children to women who are not married or have no male partners.

While artificial insemination has been practiced since the late 18th century, donor semen was apparently not used until the late 19th century. The practice did not become widespread until the second half of the 20th century. In the last several decades the demand for artificial insemination has been increasing dramatically. While the nature of legal and social problems surrounding the procedure has meant that careful records have not been kept and therefore frequency cannot be determined precisely, it has been estimated by responsible researchers that from 6000 to 20,000 A.I.D. children are born in the United States each year, and approximately one million children born as a consequence of A.I.D. are now living throughout the world.[2]

Legal Considerations

A number of legal questions are raised by the procedure of A.I.D. Persons contemplating the procedure need to be aware of the possible legal ramifications of their actions. Unfortunately, a survey of the literature reveals considerable legal confusion and contradiction in relation to artificial insemination, making predictions about court rulings very difficult.

One of the legal questions related to A.I.D. is whether or not the procedure constitutes adultery. The issue has generally been raised in connection with divorce or support proceedings. Early cases in the United States, Canada, and England held that the practice of A.I.D. was equivalent to adultery, and therefore provided grounds for divorce. The central question "is whether or not adultery requires a sexual act or whether it encompasses any action giving rise to the possibility of illegitimate conception."[3] An early Canadian case, decided by the Ontario Supreme Court, took the position that A.I.D. is adulterous because "the essence of the offense of adultery consists, not in the moral turpitude of the act of sexual intercourse, but in the voluntary surrender to another person of the reproductive powers or faculties."[4]

The practice of A.I.D. was not common when most of the adultery laws were written. In most cases, courts have held that adultery requires actual sexual intercourse. "Today it seems doubtful that any American court would hold that A.I.D. constitutes adultery."[5]

More thorny questions surround the issue of legitimacy. The concept of legitimacy is crucial in our legal system, because it bears on questions of inheritance, child support, and custody and visitation privileges. In 1964 Georgia was the first state to enact a law creating a legal presumption of legitimacy for A.I.D. children when the mother and her husband have given their legal consent to the procedure.[6] A number of other states have enacted similar statutes.

The issue has not been decided consistently, however:

> Many courts have held that a child born by AID is illegitimate without giving any regard to whether or not the husband gave his consent. . . . Practically, however, it is hard to prove

that an AID child is illegitimate. First and foremost is the fact that most states have a statute providing a *rebuttable* presumption that a child born within a marriage is the legitimate issue of that marriage. Such a presumption can be rebutted only by clear and convincing evidence that the husband is not the father. Barring complete sterility or impotency of the husband such a presumption is difficult to rebut.[7]

The concept of legitimacy is very important with reference to inheritance. Legitimate children possess the power to inherit from both their father and mother. In the case of A.I.D., the question arises whether the child can inherit from the mother's husband, who is not the biological father. Or does the child have the right to inherit from the sperm donor, assuming that paternity could be demonstrated? If the child should die before his or her parents, who then has the right to inherit according to the intestate laws of the various states? The issues of inheritance require careful legal attention by the parties involved.

Another issue associated with legitimacy has to do with child support. In case of divorce, is the mother's husband liable for the support of a child conceived by A.I.D.? Does it make a difference, legally, whether or not he consented to the procedure? When these questions have been raised, it appears that the courts have regularly held that when the husband has consented to A.I.D., he is liable for child support.[8]

The matter of custody and visitation privileges may also hinge on the legitimacy question in disputed cases. Fairness would seem to dictate that if the husband possesses the same legal duties as a natural parent in terms of child support, then he should enjoy the same legal rights in terms of custody and visitation privileges. In any event, the key consideration in such cases should be the best interests of the child.

Still another legal consideration involves the responsibility and legal liability of the doctor. The physician normally assumes a unique role in A.I.D., inasmuch as he or she selects the donor and evaluates the couple seeking this procedure. At a minimum, of course, doctors are required to exercise the degree of skill and learning common to members of the medical profession in good standing.

Since there is danger of transmitting certain infectious and genetic diseases through A.I.D., there appears to be a potential legal liability for negligence on the part of the doctor if proper screening and testing procedures are not carried out. Under a theory of strict liability, the doctor could be held responsible for using genetically defective semen.[9] In most places, however, the standards for genetic screening or testing in relation to A.I.D. are not well established.

Allen R. Moritz and C. Joseph Stetler, in their *Handbook of Legal Medicine,* have recommended that physicians should establish written agreements with the parties involved in order to avoid litigation. Such agreements, they say, should cover the following points: ''(1) written consent of the wife, including permission for the physician to use his best judgment in donor selection; (2) written consent of the husband; and (3) written consent of the donor for unrestricted use of semen. This consent can be endorsed by the donor's wife.''[10]

There remains considerable doubt, however, about the effectiveness of such written agreements:

> On its face, a consent form would seem to operate as a complete defense to any action against the doctor for negligence or strict liability. However, it is extremely doubtful that the courts would give such effect to a consent form. While these forms have not been tested in the courts in an AID case, they have been tested in other kinds of cases and found invalid. The general rule is that such consent forms are ineffective because persons may not contract away their own negligence.[11]

At best, written consent may serve to establish the intent of the parties at the time the agreement is executed.[12] The questionable benefits of such consent forms serve to underscore again the legal uncertainties that currently pervade the performance of A.I.D.

Psychological and Social Considerations

Any careful examination of the practice of A.I.D. requires that attention be given to certain psychological and social considerations. These psychological and social factors are collectively of more importance for the process of decision making than are the legal considerations discussed above.

A.I.D. offers certain potential psychological benefits over the alternative of adoption. Both husband and wife can be involved in the pregnancy from conception onward, sharing the experience of delivery and the early days of the baby's life. There is a greater chance that the child's physical appearance will at least match that of the mother, and, if there are several children, they are more likely to resemble one another. There need be no subconscious fear of the sudden appearance of the natural mother, as there may be in adoption. And, of course, the desire on the part of the mother to carry a child is satisfied as it cannot be in adoption.[13]

However, A.I.D. also poses psychological dangers to the wife, the husband, and the child. In the more usual situation of procreation by husband and wife, the child can be understood to be the joint issue of both parents. Both husband and wife fulfill for the other the opportunity to become father and mother. Their love for one another can be strengthened and deepened as a consequence of this mutually shared experience.

In the case of A.I.D., however, the situation can be very different. The wife may have a feeling of having been "cheated" by the discovery of the husband's infertility. The desire to procreate despite this discovery may become, in part, an act of revenge or hostility toward the sterile husband.[14] If A.I.D. is successful, the wife may sense that the new life she bears within her has no relation to the love she has for her husband.[15] She may, in fact, secretly yearn to meet the man who has "helped" her when the husband could not.[16]

The husband likewise faces certain psychological dangers. He may feel a stranger to the new life developing in his wife's womb. His masculinity may be threatened, not only by his infertility, but by the sense of inadequacy in comparison to the donor who made possible his wife's pregnancy. "A.I.D. thus threatens to evoke very deep-seated feelings of helpless dependence in relationship to women and also feelings of inadequacy in relation to other men."[17] The husband may psychologically withdraw from the home, investing his energy in his work or other forms of self-achievement by which he may hope to resecure his sense of masculinity.[18]

These psychological dangers for husband and wife also threaten the psychological development of the child. The child may subtly become aware of a family secret involving his or her father. If the psychological dangers for husband and wife materialize, the child may find himself or herself alienated from the father, creating another set of psychological difficulties for the child.

Closely aligned to this psychological danger is the matter of dealing with the child's genealogy. Like adoption in an earlier age, A.I.D. is usually maintained as a secret among the parties involved. The doctor, the husband and wife, and the donor conspire together to deceive the child and society regarding the child's genetic identity. George J. Annas has described the predicament in these terms:

Because of the current secrecy surrounding the practice of Artificial Insemination Donor (AID), there are an estimated

250,000 children conceived by AID. . .who will never be able
to find their biological roots. There is almost no data available
on these children, their psychological development, or their
family life. The entire procedure has been shrouded in secrecy
that is primarily justified by fear of potential legal consequences
should the fact of AID be discovered.[19]

Several arguments can be offered in favor of disclosing his
or her true genealogy to the child. In the first place, the risk
of accidental disclosure or suspicion may cause parent to decide
that forthrightly telling the child at an appropriate age would
contribute to a healthier relationship. This is similar to an argument for disclosure of adoption. It recognizes the fundamental importance of truth for basic human relationships.

An argument can also be made on the basis of the child's
right to know his or her genealogical heritage. Experience with
adopted children in recent years has shown the significance of
this knowledge of genealogical heritage for dealing with the
problem of identity as the child matures. Certainly in cases
where the child is told that he or she was conceived through
A.I.D., that child will be likely to pursue the quest for a knowledge of his or her genetic heritage. With the current inadequate
practices of record keeping, that knowledge will probably not
be available.

A final argument in favor of disclosure, and the kind of
record keeping that would make disclosure meaningful, is that
knowledge of one's genealogical heritage may be crucial if the
child suffers any genetic illness or needs a reliable family medical history. Moreover, genetic counseling at some point in the
child's life—an increasingly useful tool in preventative medicine—can be critically skewed if the child does not know his
or her paternal genealogy or, what is more likely, if the assumed paternal genealogy is not the true one.

There are, of course, a number of arguments against disclosing either the fact of A.I.D. or the identity of the donor. Some of these arguments pertain to the desire to maintain healthy family relationships, which the stigma of A.I.D. might disrupt. Lucinda Ann Smith has expressed some of these concerns:

> Knowledge by the public of a family's use of artificial insemination might be especially harmful to the acting father, as the need to utilize the artificial insemination technique implies sterility. Furthermore, just as the adopting parents often resent disclosure of the identity of the biological parents, since this disclosure can threaten their sense of parenthood, the acting father of an artificial insemination child may have the same need to preserve his sense of fatherhood. Moreover, the parents in the adoption case often are concerned that disclosure of the biological parent's identity would disrupt the development of a healthy, stable relationship between themselves and the adoptee. This concern applies with equal force in the artificial insemination context.[20]

Other arguments against disclosure are more concerned about protecting the anonymity of the donor. A study among physician practitioners of A.I.D., conducted by Curie-Cohen, Luttrell, and Shapiro, indicated that this was the primary concern for nondisclosure by the doctors:

> Central to the issue of confidentiality is anonymity of the donor. Respondents were concerned about this issue for several reasons. Donor anonymity allegedly protects the donor, the child and the parents from excessive emotional stress. Anonymity also protects the donor from legal involvement in the legitimacy and inheritance rights of children born through artificial insemination—issues that are not completely resolved. . . . Finally, doctors who have difficulty in obtaining donors promise anonymity to encourage donors to participate.

Respondents usually guaranteed donor anonymity by intentionally keeping inadequate records or by inseminating patients with multiple donors in a single cycle, making the identity of the genetic father uncertain. Respondents justified these practices in the light of recent court orders to open the records of adoption agencies.[21]

A middle way exists, whereby records containing pertinent genetic information could be kept and made available to the child at an appropriate time and under appropriate circumstances, while not disclosing the identity of the donor. Such a procedure, of course, would meet only some of the objections of those who argue the need for disclosure of the child's genealogical heritage.

Another social consideration closely related to the concern for genealogical or genetic heritage has to do with the possibility of unwitting incest between half-siblings. The concern is that A.I.D. children of the same donor may fall in love and marry. The chances of this occurring, of course, are affected by the number of times a single donor may be used. The study by Curie-Cohen et al., reported in the *New England Journal of Medicine* shows that some doctors use the same donor over and over. Many of the doctors used the same donor for more than six conceptions, and 10.3% of those responding used the same donor for an average of nine or more pregnancies.[22] Considering the fact that semen from the same donor is often used with women who live in the same geographic community and who may represent a rather homogeneous ethnic or social group, the possibility of incest, though small, is not farfetched.

Another issue of social significance in considering the practice of A.I.D. concerns the small but apparently growing number of unmarried women who are seeking artificial insemination as a way of becoming mothers. The study by Curie-Cohen et al. indicated that at least 9.5% of the doctors responding had used A.I.D. for single women.[23] The acceptance of "bachelor mothers" appears to be a growing trend in our society. The issue becomes even more complex when A.I.D. is used by lesbian couples, and the resulting child grows up to discover that both of his or her "parents" are female! Such developments clearly deal a serious blow to the child and to our accepted understanding of the family as the basic unit of our society.

Finally, A.I.D. also involves eugenic considerations. The attempt to influence the genetic quality of the human species by carefully selecting donors is probably never completely absent from the procedure. Negative eugenics—to prevent the birth of a potentially defective child—is certainly involved when A.I.D. is used explicitly to avoid transmitting genetic defects of the husband. Negative eugenics also provides the logical rationale for genetic screening of donors, in an attempt to reduce the risk of transmitting disease. The Curie-Cohen et al. study showed, however, that donors usually are subjected to very little genetic screening. The screening that is done often reflects a wholly inadequate understanding of rudimentary genetic principles.[24] Nevertheless, the principle of negative eugenics provides few ethical problems per se, if A.I.D. is acceptable on other grounds.

Positive eugenics (designing a reproductive program to "improve" the human race) raises more serious questions. At an informal level a certain kind of positive eugenics inheres in the usual practice of doctors selecting medical students or hospital residents as donors. Annas has put the matter clearly:

> There can be little debate that physicians in all of these situations are making eugenic decisions—selecting what they consider "superior" genes for AID. In general they have chosen to reproduce themselves (or those in their profession), and this is what sociobiologists would probably have predicted. . . .

Physicians may believe that society needs more individuals with the attributes of physicians, but it is unlikely that society as a whole does. Lawyers would be likely to select law students; geneticists, graduate students in genetics; military personnel, students at the military academies, and so on.[25]

Be that as it may, one need not see in this practice a genetic plot on the part of physicians, since the practice of selecting medical students or hospital residents as donors is undoubtedly motivated largely by convenience.

Far more insidious are the attempts to organize sperm banks for the purpose of improving the human race through carefully selected genetic material. The most famous—or infamous—of these is the Nobel sperm bank established in California, which accepts only men who have won the Nobel Prize in science as donors. Its defenders advocate a kind of selective breeding that aspires toward the development of a super race.[26] Such peddling of "celebrity seed" raises profound questions about what human qualities should be considered "desirable," and about who should or will make such decisions in our society.

Ethical Considerations

None of the foregoing considerations are without ethical significance. However, it is my contention that the chief ethical issue, on which hinges one's ultimate decision for or against A.I.D., has to do with the nature of marriage and parenthood. This is the issue that finally underlies our ethical assessment of many of the other considerations discussed above. What is the nature of the marriage bond, and what significance does this have for our assessment of A.I.D.? What is the proper relationship between this marriage bond and the procreation of children? These are the crucial ethical questions in determining our decisions about A.I.D.

Contemporary ethicists have taken widely disparate views of these questions. Joseph Fletcher, the father of "situation ethics," takes a view that does not see the marital bond as necessitating a physical monopoly. He stresses the "personal" character of the marriage covenant and goes on to assert that since no personal relationship is entered into with the donor, A.I.D. is acceptable when mutually agreed upon by husband and wife. In such a case there is no broken faith, no infidelity, between them.

Fletcher summarizes his views:

> We have asserted two things, fundamentally: (1) that the fidelity of marriage is a *personal* bond between husband and wife, not primarily a legal contract, and (2) that parenthood is a *moral* relationship with children, not a material or merely physical relationship. The claim that A.I.D. is immoral rests upon the view that marriage is an absolute generative, as well as sexual, monopoly; and that parenthood is an essentially, if not solely, physiological partnership. Neither of these ideas is compatible with a morality that welcomes emancipation from natural necessity, or with the Christian ethic which raises morality to the level of love (a *personal* bond), above the determinism of nature and the rigidities of law as distinguished from love.[27]

In characteristic fashion Fletcher finds love and law incompatible and insists that rules are less than Christian. And he asserts that "to transcend natural restrictions, to seek ends by means devised through choice rather than by physical determinism, is a human and spiritual victory. With many of us it is a matter of reasoned conviction that our march toward freedom and control is an irreversible trend."[28] Thus Fletcher puts an emphasis on the "personal" character of the marriage bond rather than on any notion of a physical bond. He is unfettered by notions of the rightness or wrongness of given physical acts apart from the meaning love assigns to them. And he exalts the victory of the spiritual over the physical in the opportunities for choice offered through the technology of A.I.D. He therefore celebrates this option when it is mutually agreed upon by husband and wife.

An altogether different view is set forth by Paul Ramsey. Ramsey examines the nature of the marriage bond and argues that the marriage bond and procreation are inseparable. He contends that A.I.D. divides the sexual unity between husband and wife and therefore violates the covenant of marriage.

Ramsey argues that the very nature of sexual intercourse combines a unitive and a procreative function:

> An act of sexual intercourse is at the same time an act of love and a procreative act. This does not mean that sexual intercourse always in fact nourishes love between the parties or always engenders a child. It simply means that it *tends*, of its own nature, toward the strengthening of love (the unitive or the communitive good), and toward the engendering of children (the procreative good).[29]

Since God has placed the unitive and procreative goods together in sexual intercourse, they ought never to be put entirely asunder:

> An ethics (whether proposed by nominal Christians or not) that *in principle* sunders these two goods—regarding procreation as an aspect of biological nature to be subjected merely to the requirements of *technical* control while saying that the unitive purpose is the free, human, personal end of the matter—pays disrespect to the nature of human parenthood. *Human* parenthood is not the same as that of the animals God gave Adam complete dominion over.[30]

Ramsey does not argue against contraception. People can practice responsible birth control without separating the sphere or realm of their personal love from the sphere or realm of their procreation. The person with whom the bond of love is nourished and the person with whom procreation is exercised remains the same. Though contraception is practiced with regard to a particular act or particular acts of sexual intercourse, the totality of such sexual acts by a married couple holds together the unitive and procreative goods. "Where planned parenthood is not planned *un*parenthood, the husband and wife clearly do not tear their own one-flesh unity completely away from all positive response and obedience to the mystery of procreation—a power by which at a later time their own union originates the one flesh of a child."[31]

Even in a marriage in which a responsible decision has been made to have no children, the unitive and procreative functions of sexual intercourse are honored. The marriage partners still concur by the nature of their commitment that *if* either of the partners has a child, it will be "within their marriage-covenant, from their own one-flesh unity and not apart from it."[32] Ramsey concludes that practicing birth control, even lifelong birth control, does not divide the unitive and procreative functions of sexual intercourse for a married couple, because "they do not procreate from beyond their marriage, or exercise love's one-flesh unity elsewhere."[33]

At least in part, Ramsey derives his insistence that the fundamental oneness of the unitive and procreative nature of sexual intercourse within marriage should not be bypassed from his reading of the prolog of John and Ephesians 5. It is in this connection that he states his position most succinctly:

> We procreate new beings like ourselves in the midst of our love for one another, and in this there is a trace of the original mystery by which God created the world because of His love. God created nothing apart from His love; and without the divine love was not anything made that was made. Neither should

there be among men and women (whose man-womanhood—
and not their minds or wills only—is in the image of God) any
love set out of the context of responsibility for procreation,
any begetting apart from the sphere of love. A reflection of
God's love, binding himself to the world and the world to
himself, is found in the claim He placed upon men and women
in their creation when He bound the nurturing of marital love
and procreation together in the nature of human sexuality. . . .
To put radically asunder what God joined together in parenthood when He made love procreative, to procreate from beyond
the sphere of love (AID, for example . . .), or to posit acts
of sexual love beyond the sphere of responsible procreation
(by definition, marriage), means a refusal of the image of God's
creation in our own.[34]

A.I.D. is rejected because the personal and the physical
cannot be separated without dividing what God has put together
in the very nature of sexual intercourse. In A.I.D. the nature
of human parenthood is assaulted by putting the bodily transmission of life completely asunder from bodily lovemaking.
A.I.D. is therefore contrary to God's intention that children
should be the fruit of the loving gift of husband and wife to
one another.

Helmut Thielicke argues against A.I.D. on similar grounds.
He states that "the problem is presented by the fact that here
a third person enters into the exclusive psychophysical relationship of marriage, even though it is only his sperm that
'represents' him."[35] The introduction of donor semen therefore
violates the *mysterium* of marital fellowship, the psychophysical unity of husband and wife. "This violation also manifests
itself when the fulfillment of motherhood which is not accompanied by the fulfillment of fatherhood breaks down the personal solidarity of the married couple."[36] Even if the husband
consents to the procedure, psychic and physical realities are

called into play that have a life of their own, despite his initial motivation. A.I.D. is therefore rejected.

Harmon Smith also expounds a position rejecting A.I.D. for reasons much like those offered by Ramsey and Thielicke. He reasons that procreation must always spring from the love of a couple, which constitutes the very core of the marriage bond:

> I have argued that human procreation, Christianly understood, differs from animal or plant procreation precisely in the measure to which it functions within, and in order to incarnate, an antecedent loving relationship. I have argued, moreover, that on this understanding the two inseparable goods of human sexuality are disunited when procreation occurs from beyond the sphere of love or when acts of sexual love occur from beyond the sphere of willingness to be responsible for procreation.[37]

> AID separates procreation from love in the measure to which neither donor nor recipient posits his or her act within the sphere of a love which unites them. In AID each functions, as it were, from ''outside'' the other, thereby putting asunder ''what God joined together'' when he made love procreative.[38]

It should be noted that the arguments of Ramsey, Thielicke, and Smith are directed against A.I.D. and do not apply to artificial insemination by the husband.

Roman Catholic theologians, in the main, have also rejected A.I.D. A number of secondary arguments are adduced against the practice, dealing with such matters as the immorality of masturbation as it is understood within the framework of traditional Roman Catholic moral theology. None of these secondary arguments appear to be insurmountable, however.

The primary reason for Roman Catholic opposition to A.I.D. is that it removes procreation from within the marriage bond. The official position of the Roman Catholic church was stated

by Pope Pius XII in 1949. After condemning artificial insemination outside of marriage, he went on to reject A.I.D. within
marriage as well:

> Artificial insemination in marriage with the use of an active
> element from a third person is equally immoral and as such is
> to be rejected summarily. Only the marriage partners have
> mutual rights over their bodies for the procreation of a new
> life and these are exclusive, non-transferable and inalienable
> rights. So it must be, out of consideration for the child.
>
> By virtue of this same bond, nature imposes on whoever
> gives life to a small creature the task of its preservation and
> education. Between the marriage partners, however, and a
> child which is the fruit of the active element of a third person—
> even though the husband consents—there is no bond of origin,
> no moral or juridical bond of conjugal procreation.[39]

A.I.D. is thus understood as contrary to the divine plan for
marriage and parenthood. It is an essentially disordered act.

Karl Rahner, a leading Roman Catholic theologian, has put
it this way:

> Now this personal love which is consummated sexually has
> within it an essential inner relation to the child, for the child
> is an embodiment of the abiding unity of the marriage partners
> which is expressed in marital union. Genetic manipulation [by
> which Rahner means A.I.D.], however, does two things: it
> fundamentally separates the marital union from the procreation
> of a new person as this permanent embodiment of the unity of
> married love; and it transfers procreation, isolated and torn
> from its human matrix, to an area outside man's sphere of
> intimacy. It is this sphere of intimacy which is the proper
> context for sexual union, which itself implies the fundamental
> readiness of the marriage-partners to let their unity take the
> form of a child.[40]

Reflections/Conclusions

On the basis of the foregoing discussion, what reflections can be offered and what conclusions drawn with respect to the practice of A.I.D.? In my opinion A.I.D. is not an ethically acceptable alternative to childlessness in the case of male infertility. Several fundamental considerations lead to this conclusion.

Though not absolutely determinative from an ethical viewpoint, the psychological dangers described above weigh heavily against a decision to employ A.I.D. The radical asymmetry of the parents' relationship to the A.I.D. child opens the door to a host of psychological difficulties. It should be acknowledged that in theory, of course, these psychological difficulties are not insurmountable. But they appear sufficiently grave to compel extreme caution.

More serious from an ethical standpoint is the moral assessment of the role played by the donor. Though not explicitly dealt with in the ethical considerations discussed above, that discussion does bear implicitly on the donor's responsibility for his actions. The donor clearly exercises his procreative powers apart from any marital bond or commitment. He remains anonymously hidden from both the mother and the child, refusing his responsibility as father. His function remains that of a sperm salesman, failing to take full responsibility for his biological offspring. Even though it may be argued that he acts out of love to provide a child for a childless couple, nevertheless love can never oblige one to perform an action which by its nature violates the fundamental unity of the personal and biological dimensions of sexual intercourse within the covenant of marriage.

It is the nature of the marital covenant and the meaning of parenthood that provides the critical norm for judging the fundamental ethical stance toward A.I.D. With the majority of ethicists cited above I argue that marriage is a deeply personal commitment in which husband and wife mutually confer exclusive fidelity to one another, which includes the mutual commitment of procreative powers. By the introduction of donor semen, A.I.D. separates procreation from marriage and thereby violates the marriage covenant.

Those who offer contrary arguments in favor of A.I.D. explicitly or implicitly separate the personal from the physical, the unitive from the procreative function of the sex act. They thus fall prey to the destructive dualism that has plagued Western culture, whereby the personal or spiritual is understood as the specifically human and the physical or bodily is frequently depreciated. The personal is too readily understood as a disembodied spiritual reality.

I would argue that we cannot separate the meaning of "personal" and "human" from physical, bodily processes. Ramsey is right when he contends:

> We need rather the biblical comprehension that man is as much the body of his soul as he is the soul of his body. The single word *sarx* in the "one-flesh" unity of marriage and parenthood is sufficient to impel us to think with the Jews and Christians in all ages who have affirmed a unity between the vocations of soul and body. They therefore affirmed the biological to be *assumed into* the personal and in some ultimate sense believed there is a linkage between the love-making and the life-giving "dimensions" of this one-flesh unity of ours.[41]

Only when this unity is maintained can children be understood in the full sense as the visible fruit and extension of conjugal love.

A.I.D. cannot be ethically accepted simply because, like other good technologies, it "works," that is, because it gives a child to a childless couple. From the standpoint of ethics we need to be concerned not only about right ends, but also about correct means. And in this case, the means violate the fundamental meaning of sexual intercourse within the covenant of marriage. Even when the husband consents, ''AID signifies less than an unreserved commitment to share another's life 'for better or worse, in sickness and in health.' ''[42]

None of these ethical objections should be construed, of course, in such a way as to cast a moral shadow on the child who has been so conceived. Nor does A.I.D. fall into the category of some unforgivable sin. But on the basis of the above considerations, a couple who find themselves childless because of male infertility are better advised either to come to terms with their childlessness or to seek children through adoption.

On Having Children: A Theological and Moral Analysis of *In Vitro* Fertilization

—————— *Paul T. Jersild* ——————

The advances in technology during the last few decades have created moral issues that were hardly imagined by previous generations. This is strikingly true in the area of medical technology. Here the advances have radically altered the boundaries both of birth and death. Far more human sovereignty is now exercised over nascent life and the process of dying, with the result that we now have options that involve our *choosing* between life and death. Thus both abortion and euthanasia have moved to the forefront as critical social issues.

In vitro fertilization (IVF), unlike abortion and euthanasia, does not refer to the termination of human life. It describes a procedure by which life is facilitated through human manipulation, and as such it increases further our sovereignty over the genesis of fellow human beings. IVF simply intensifies the fundamental question raised by advances in medical technology: who are we as human beings? Because it raises this basic question, IVF deserves careful theological and moral analysis in order to determine whether it is a procedure that ultimately serves our humanity or possibly destroys it. Our purpose here is to examine that question and arrive at an answer that appears to be responsible in view of Christian conviction.

IVF as a Medical and Therapeutic Procedure

Historical Background

The possibility of fertilizing an egg in an artificial environment (*in vitro* means literally "in glass," or in a laboratory dish outside of the body) has fascinated the medical community for some time. An unsuccessful attempt was made in Germany in 1878 to fertilize eggs in the laboratory. The same experiment met with success in 1934. Ten years later John Rock of Harvard University reported success in fertilizing the human egg with sperm *in vitro,* and Landrum Shettles of Columbia University did the same in 1953. To prove that the fertilization occurring *in vitro* was genuine, M. C. Chang of the Worcester Foundation of Experimental Biology in 1959 inserted a fertilized rabbit egg into the womb of a second female rabbit, resulting in pregnancy. By 1969 it was clear that the necessary techniques for IVF were available.

The first human pregnancy induced through IVF occurred in Melbourne, Australia, in 1973, but it lasted only nine days. In England, Robert Edwards and Patrick Steptoe had developed the technique known as laparoscopy, which enabled a more successful retrieval of the woman's eggs. They also perfected the IVF procedure by injecting hormones to cause the ovary to superovulate. With more than one egg per month, chances for success were now enhanced.

The successful outcome of these developments occurred in England on July 25, 1978, with the birth of Louise Brown, the first so-called "test-tube baby." This success was followed in Australia in 1980 and in the United States in 1981. Requests for IVF on the part of infertile couples now grew by the thousands. The number of IVF clinics both here and abroad was close to 100 by mid-1983, and the number of IVF babies was nearing 200 (including at least 22 in the United States). It is estimated that by the end of 1984 there will be more than 2000 IVF babies in the world, at least 200 of them in the United States. The future appears to promise IVF as a fairly routine procedure in overcoming the burden of childlessness.

Childlessness in Our Society

It is not difficult to perceive why childlessness can be a burden to a couple, and particularly to the woman. Historically the principal role of women has been to bear and nurture children. For the Christian community this tradition goes back to the Old Testament, in which the woman was regarded as failing her husband and the divine command to "be fruitful and multiply" if she had the misfortune to be childless. The absence of children was associated with divine disfavor. The New Testament did not materially alter this kind of thinking, except that the coming of the kingdom of God received precedence even over marriage and family life. Thus the possibility of celibacy as a response to the kingdom became an acceptable vocation in the Christian tradition.

Roman Catholicism has consistently maintained that marriage and children are indissolubly linked, leading to the rejection of any artificial means of birth control. Protestantism regards children as desirable and a blessing, but defines marriage primarily in terms of the covenant between two persons. In the context of recent developments in our society an increasing number of theologians have concluded that voluntary childlessness is conceivable for a Christian couple, and that the absence of children does not prevent a full and complete marriage relationship. This is a logical corollary to the view expressed in the current women's movement, which has enlarged the vision of female vocation to embrace not just the home and family but the marketplace as well. Indeed, many have argued that a woman must find it difficult if not impossible to arrive at self-fulfillment within her traditional role of mothering.

In view of these sociological developments which are liberating the woman from the home, it is interesting that IVF now becomes a coveted option for childless couples.[1] Just at the time when childlessness is becoming intelligible and acceptable as a choice for many couples, medical technology promises a child to those who are without. The desire to have one's own child remains strong in spite of changing mores concerning the desirability of children.

The experience of couples in facing their infertility can be exceedingly painful. It can be experienced as a great void, the source of a fundamentally incomplete life. Adopting a child has been the alternative for many in this predicament, but others have not found this to be satisfactory. Having a child ''of one's own'' is seen as more than having an adopted child. The desire is to have a child who is ''flesh of my flesh,'' a desire perhaps complicated in some cases by feelings of inadequacy or even abnormality concerning one's infertility. The pain, inconvenience, and humiliating procedures that are patiently borne by couples—particularly the woman—in their efforts to have their own child are ample evidence of the strength of this desire. For these couples, IVF has now become the final option, promising success after years of much frustration and often deep despair.

It is not known just how many couples are potential beneficiaries of IVF. In testimony before the Ethics Advisory

Board of HEW, John D. Biggers roughly estimated the upper limits of need in the United States as follows:

> There are 60 million women reproductively active in the USA; seven percent of couples are infertile, and a third of these are infertile because of sterility of the wife. Thus, there are 1,400,000 sterile women in the population.[2]

IVF is not the answer in every instance of infertility, but it is a possible answer under such circumstances as the following:

1. When the fallopian tubes, which link the ovaries with the uterus, are diseased or blocked. This is the common reason for IVF; according to Biggers' estimate there are some 560,000 women with diseased oviducts.

2. When the husband's sperm are abnormal, either in number, movement, or structure, and fail to respond to treatment. In the controlled environment of IVF, some of these problems can be overcome.

3. When the reason for infertility is unknown, which accounts for close to 10% of cases of infertility. This includes the possibility that there are undetected abnormalities in the eggs or sperm, or other factors which inhibit fertilization.

The Medical Procedure

In preparing for IVF, a woman is given hormones for five to seven days to stimulate growth of ova (eggs) within the follicles in the ovaries. Another hormone injection controls the precise time, 32 hours later, when the eggs are ready for removal. This precise timing makes it possible to have a full medical staff in readiness. A small incision is made near the navel, and a miniature viewing device with a light, called a laparoscope, is inserted in order to give the physician a picture of the internal organs and the collection of eggs. A hollow needle is used to suck the egg cell from its nest, or follicle, on the surface of the ovary. Timing is critical, for the egg cannot be used if it is fully ripe and ejected before removal, or if it is not quite mature enough. The eggs remain in their follicular fluid, and relatively little damage occurs; about 10% of them are lost in this procedure.

The eggs are allowed to mature by waiting five or six hours before they are exposed in a dish to about 100,000 sperm. During the next 40 to 60 hours the fertilized eggs develop into four- or eight-cell embryos. At this point they are ready to be implanted in the woman's uterus. This is called an embryo transfer, in which one or more embryos, hardly visible to the naked eye, are transferred in a transparent plastic tube through the vagina and cervix into the uterus. To maximize the possibility that at least one embryo will implant in the uterine wall, the woman must remain in bed for about 18 hours.

The chances for a successful pregnancy are not high. It is generally estimated that one out of five embryos will be successfully implanted and result in a normal pregnancy. At the Eastern Virginia Medical School in Norfolk, where IVF was first successfully performed in the United States, the success rate has been just 10% when one embryo is transferred. This rate has increased to approximately 50% with the transfer of three embryos. Though running a small ''risk'' of multiple births, most couples understandably prefer multiple transfers in order to increase the possibility of success.

The medical procedure is not particularly complicated, nor is it of any great risk to the woman. Its intent is laudable enough in enabling a couple to have their own child. As we turn to theological and moral considerations, we must focus on certain aspects of the procedure not yet discussed, as well as possible variations of the procedure that raise serious questions for many concerning the appropriateness of IVF.

Theological and Moral Considerations

Raising the Theological Question

Though some continue to believe so, there is no divine information from which theologians can pull an indisputable answer to the question of IVF. Those with a fundamentalist orientation are easily tempted to believe that a particular passage from the Bible can provide a conclusive and authoritative answer to a particular social issue. This invariably results in a manipulation of Scripture that simply expresses the particular bias of the individual. It betrays the desire for simplistic solutions to complicated problems and turns the Scripture into an arbitrary handbook. The matter becomes yet more ambiguous when one is addressing dilemmas created by an advanced technology or situations never imagined by the biblical writers.

The initial concern of theologians must be to inform themselves as extensively as possible concerning the nature of a given issue. This is an empirical task, determining the facts of the matter, as well as an interpretive task, understanding its full dimensions and significance. Methodological tools and insights from the social sciences are an indispensable resource here. When this task has been responsibly addressed, the Christian theologian will seek guidance from Scripture and the larger tradition. This guidance may come in several ways, involving both moral insight (from principles and paradigms emerging from the variety of biblical material) and theological perspective, but a fundamental concern will be to relate the context of ultimate meaning for the human story proclaimed in Scripture to the particular issue one is addressing. This presents a challenging hermeneutical task.

Rather than moving directly from isolated scripture passages to a particular social issue, the theologian's task is first to determine the theological truths that capture the essential meaning of the scriptural revelation. One's theological tradition will provide an orientation in carrying out this task, and the tradition itself may bring a perspective that will shape one's attitude toward a given social issue. In making this connection between theological conviction and responsible behavior, it is helpful to determine what questions the issue itself raises for faith. In regard to IVF, Stanley Hauerwas suggests that the appropriate question is, "Why have children?"[3] In other words, IVF challenges the Christian theologian to reflect on the meaning and purpose of childbearing in light of the Christian message. One can think of a variety of possible answers to why we have children (to enjoy them, to have their support when we need them, to continue the race, to continue our own lineage), but from a Christian stance the ultimate answer is because we believe in God—that is, we have hope in the future of humanity, and we accept our parenthood as a stewardship from God.

Parenthood involves both the procreative dimension (childbearing) and the much more multifaceted dimension of nurture and care (childrearing). It is this latter area which defines the essential task and responsibility of parenthood before God and the community. Childbearing is simply the prelude to the major work of childrearing, where faith, hope, and love are daily exercised and challenged. In nurturing the child the parents are presenting their "gift" from God as their own gift to the kingdom and to the community (a truth that does not deny the growing independence of the child as he or she moves beyond the authority of the parents, but recognizes the critical foundation laid by the parents in the development of the child). Here is where the real meaning of parenthood from a Christian perspective is to be found, rather than in the experience of childbearing.

The inference to be drawn from this understanding is neither a total rejection nor total acceptance of IVF. It does imply, however, that the procedure ought not be a high priority for parents desiring children. Parenthood before God is not fundamentally defined by its biology but by its nurture. IVF provides the experience of pregnancy and the satisfaction of having a child "of one's own flesh," desires that are understandable and not to be treated lightly. But they are not essential to the responsibility and blessings of parenthood. This means that the desire on the part of infertile couples to have their own child will have to be weighed in relation to other needs and resources of the community. It is not a right, nor even essential to the role of parenting.

Other theological views found in the Christian community result in different conclusions regarding IVF. For example, the tradition of natural law maintains a God-given order in the structures of human life that ought not be compromised by our technology. It is concerned to recognize proper limits to human manipulation of nature, limits transgressed only at our peril. In regard to human reproduction, the limitations are implicit in the natural order of procreation, in which the embrace of conjugal love is united with the conceiving of new life. Since IVF ruptures this unity with the intrusion of the laboratory, it challenges divine wisdom and paves the way for further aberrations in human reproduction. Thus the traditional Roman Catholic view, rooted in a natural-law tradition, consistently rejects both contraception (sex without babies) and IVF (babies without sex). As early as 1949 Pope Pius XII rejected any attempt to facilitate conception apart from the sexual act as "immoral" and "absolutely illicit."

Others argue on theological grounds for the appropriateness of IVF. They note that the biblical story reveals a God of history who is not identified with a static, eternal order of nature but beckons his people into a changing future. Rather than finding the moral imperative in apparent structures of a social order, we should be intent on exercising our God-given imagination and technological skills to create a more humane world. IVF is an achievement to be welcomed because it reduces human pain and opens the future for infertile couples locked in the despair of childlessness. Only if the end results of IVF constitute a clear threat to human welfare should it be prohibited.

Arriving at a Moral Evaluation

The moral arguments for and against IVF tend to proceed either from principles based on the nature of procreation, with their implications for IVF, or on anticipated effects of the procedure and an evaluation of those effects. These two approaches reflect traditional methods of arriving at moral judgments. The one argues that the very nature of things compels one to say that one ought or ought not to engage in a particular action (deontological argument). The conviction here is that the various human relationships embody values intrinsic to those relationships and one ought not violate them regardless how noble the intended goal of one's action. The other argument is based on the end or goal of what we do (teleological argument). Here the value of an act is determined by whether it best serves an ideal end to which other values should be subordinated. Moral reflection must be sensitive to the concerns of both of these approaches. The result may be a continuing tension between competing values that may never be resolved to one's satisfaction. Yet one finally attributes greater weight or priority to one value over another in arriving at a decision.

A first and obvious moral concern about IVF relates to the well-being of those who are born through the procedure. We are obligated to know for certain that the manipulation involved is not detrimental to them. Some ethicists question whether sufficient research at the animal level has been done to warrant the practice of IVF among humans. Possible long-term effects are still not known. If this concern has substance, IVF would constitute unethical experimentation with the yet unborn. This would also involve questions of consent regarding the unborn:

> It is one thing voluntarily to accept the risk of a dangerous procedure for yourself (or to consent on behalf of your child) if the *purpose is therapeutic*. . . . It is quite a different thing to submit a child to hazardous procedures which can in no way be therapeutic for him. . . . This argument against nontherapeutic experimentation on children applies with even greater force against experimentation "on" a hypothetical child (whose conception is as yet only intellectual). One cannot ethically choose for him the unknown hazards he must face and simultaneously choose to give him life in which to face them.[4]

Potential risk for the IVF baby remains a question of judgment, but generally the scientific community appears satisfied that reasonable and necessary precautions have been taken and that sufficient knowledge has been gained to proceed with confidence. At this point, at least, it would appear that the children conceived by IVF are happy to be here.

A further issue in assessing IVF is the seriousness of human manipulation in the process of procreation. Is the intrusion of the laboratory an inherent evil? If it destroys or in some way compromises what is perceived to be a morally desirable and even necessary relation between the parents, or between parent and child, then it would be a moral evil that ought not be allowed. But it is difficult to establish this argument on moral grounds. As we have noted, one can argue theologically for the necessary connection of procreation with the sexual act based on the notion of a "divine intendedness" to the natural order. It is not as easy, however, to demonstrate an inherent necessity to this connection on moral grounds without simply positing it as a "given," which therefore must not be destroyed. This will appear arbitrary if it is not supported by some form of consequential argument.

The feared consequence most often cited relates to the moral health of society as a whole. Does the introduction of human manipulation dehumanize the process of procreation? The initial reason for introducing human manipulation in the procreative process is praiseworthy: to enable infertile couples to have their own children. But with human intrusion other goals made achievable by technology are also introduced. This includes our gaining control over procreation in order to avoid the "chance character" and arbitrariness of human genesis. Procreation subject to human manipulation is procreation guaranteed to provide us with the end "product" we desire through careful selection of genetic traits. It raises the possibility of procreation without pain and discomfort, procreation as a servant even to whim and desire. In short, technology in the realm of procreation can be seen as ultimately dehumanizing because it subordinates human life to the values of a consumer culture. The human values of mystery and surprise give way to control, which enables prediction and the avoidance of discomfort. Procreation becomes reproduction.[5]

Joseph Fletcher argues that, to the contrary, technology is not a source of dehumanizing but the expression of human genius and therefore a humanizing resource. It is more "human," according to Fletcher, to bring a baby to term in a completely artificial environment than in the woman's womb, for to do so is the result of human creativity and purpose. The basic issue for Fletcher is whether we are willing to leave the realm of chance and gain control over the fruits of reproduction. To do so is to "exercise our rational and human choice, no longer submissively trusting to the blind worship of raw nature.''[6] Exercising control and autonomy is a good, not an evil.

And yet, the product of human genius is motivated by desires both good and bad. The quest for sovereignty over all dimenions of life, while fully human in character, is not an automatic good; it often brings destruction into the human story. We have noted the difficulty in establishing on moral grounds the obligation to adhere to a ''natural'' or given order of things, but one might counter Fletcher's position with the argument that procreation as a natural process is integral to human identity itself. While human manipulation on a limited scale (fetal surgery, for example, to correct a defect) can contribute significantly to the humanizing of life, the temptation to ''improve'' on the process of procreation may result in an assault on our self-consciousness as human beings. We are not human products, but rather the end of a creative process in which our parents are privileged to share and which is beyond the complete control of any human agency. For the sake of our humanity, then, we must carefully limit the extent of human sovereignty over such fundamental processes as those involved in human genesis. The message of *Brave New World* and other negative utopias is not to be treated lightly.

At the same time as one expresses the above concerns, one must be careful about positing a direct and inexorable movement from IVF to *Brave New World*. We may quite possibly never arrive at significant numbers of IVF patients. Furthermore, the controls exercised by clinics restrict the possibility of aberrant practices in regard to which patients are selected for treatment as well as what procedures are allowed.[7] Yet already a number of variations in the IVF procedure are occurring that raise the question of appropriate limits to the kinds of therapy offered. Infertility can be regarded as a handicap that medicine properly addresses, but the problems of infertility quickly move us beyond the established couple whose own gametes (sperm and egg) are being used. Consider the following:

1. In cases where the woman's ovaries are not functioning and it is impossible to secure an ovum (egg) of her own, it is possible to make use of the ovum of another woman. This would be the female version of A.I.D.—artificial insemination by donor—in which the sperm of another male are used when those of the husband are defective. Recently researchers at the University of California at Los Angeles successfully carried out a variation of this procedure that avoids surgery (i.e., a laparoscopy). Woman A was artificially inseminated with the sperm of woman B's husband. At the proper time the fertilized egg was flushed from her uterine cavity and implanted in the uterus of woman B. This is called an ovum transfer.

2. When the couple is incapable of providing both sperm and egg, "embryo adoption" is possible. The sperm and egg of two other persons are united *in vitro* and then implanted in the woman's uterus.

3. Should the woman be incapable of bearing her child because of a defective uterus, it is possible to implant the embryo belonging to herself and her husband in the uterus of another woman who becomes a "surrogate mother" or substitute bearer of the child. There are considerable legal complications to this practice, however.

The question these developments raise is whether IVF does not place us on a "slippery slope" that could result in serious consequences for the moral welfare of the family and society. Much of the theological and moral objection to the procedure is prompted by these variations, as well as others that are anticipated in the more distant future. Such developments, for example, as ova and embryo banks (in addition to the sperm banks already in use) are encouraged by the availability of IVF.

Supporters of IVF counter these concerns by expressing their confidence in the ability of our society to exercise appropriate restraints on the use of the procedure. They argue, furthermore, that the abuse of any life-serving procedure is no justification for discontinuing its use (*abusus non tollit usus*). Every new scientific advance involves risks; nothing would be accomplished if we were unwilling to take them. But even genuine risks can become confused with irrelevant issues in the "parade of horribles" that opponents of IVF recite in an effort to discredit it. Surrogate motherhood, for example, is not to be identified with IVF simply because it may occur in cases where the substitute is impregnated through artificial insemination. It is a matter that should be evaluated apart from IVF.

The principal reason for supporting IVF is that it makes childbearing possible for couples who desperately want their own child. This is the goal of the procedure, which to supporters more than justifies whatever risks might be associated with it. The end justifies the means. Because it is a life-serving procedure, any destructive consequences must be weighed in relation to the positive end that is attained. In weighing these consequences, however, antiabortionists usually conclude that the end in IVF does not justify the means. Because the procedure involves the discarding of embryos that are either defective or simply not needed, it is seen as necessitating abortion. Nonetheless, there are a number of factors here that lead me to believe that under appropriate control, the loss of some embryos should not in itself be reason for prohibiting IVF.

The Roman Catholic moral theologian Charles Curran contends that "truly human life is not present until two to three weeks after conception," for not until then is true individuality present beyond the possibility of twinning and recombination.[8] He calls this the "individual-biological criterion" by which to determine the beginning of human life; while it may appear to some to be a scholastic argument, it does provide a basis for making a distinction that many believe necessary between the very beginning of life in its microscopic stage and some later stage of development. This distinction is supported by the fact that under normal conditions "more than fifty percent of human conceptuses are destined to abort, many before the skipped menstrual period."[9] In other words, discarding embryos found to be defective is performing the function that takes place in spontaneous abortions. Some would insist that every healthy embryo must be implanted, while others would allow for a minimal loss. In any event it is necessary to establish restrictions that insure respect for embryonic life, without regarding each embryo as possessing a divine right to life.

Another feature in the IVF procedure that has raised apprehensions is the practice of freezing embryos in liquid nitrogen and keeping them in storage for future use. This practice enables the woman to receive a second or third embryo transfer without having to undergo additional surgery. Such freeze storage is common in cattle breeding and apparently causes no harm to the embryo. But questions inevitably remain on this score, as well as concern over the dehumanizing effects of such a practice.[10] An immediate question is whether freeze storing would be limited to facilitating the IVF procedure or would result in long-term storage to serve a variety of purposes. For example, professional couples who desire to hold off having children until their late 30s or early 40s may want to take advantage of embryo storage to avoid the higher incidence of defective embryos at that age. Such a decision would pose complications, should the couple in the meantime get a divorce.

To whom then does the embryo belong? Embryo banks designed to give childless couples the opportunity to select an embryo of their choice pose similar problems, should some embryos never be chosen. Yet such complications—and many more could be imagined—have not stopped Drs. Steptoe and Edwards from proposing an embryo bank at their clinic in England for the purpose of providing infertile couples the convenience of ''prenatal adoption.'' A similar program is operating in Melbourne, Australia.

Conclusion

The potential complications posed by IVF should be apparent to everyone who seriously considers the subject. But despite the sobering possibilities, I believe the church should not categorically reject the procedure. For the parents who are enabled to have their own child through IVF there is no sense whatever of their bearing a less than fully human and precious child. The procedure provides rich blessing for couples who in most cases have lived through a long night of despair. It is indeed a life-serving act.

At the same time, the first of the three theological positions presented above puts IVF in what I believe is a proper perspective. It should not be regarded as a high priority, but rather weighed against the considerable values of adoption. The infertile couple considering IVF should, with the help of counsel, carefully scrutinize their motivations. To have a child of one's own lineage is understandable, but it should not be an obsession that could possibly destroy the marriage if success is not achieved through IVF. Each spouse should understand that the marriage covenant, ''for better or for worse,'' encompasses also the unfortunate possibility that infertility may characterize their union.

Two additional factors should be noted in assessing the appropriateness of IVF. Within a year from the time the clinic in Norfolk opened, some 6000 had applied for its services. Only 41 could be accepted. Should the medical establishment attempt to meet this apparent demand? Does this kind of therapy warrant a major effort in time and expense on the part of our nation's medical resources? What other responsibilities of our hospitals and clinics would be neglected as a result? From my own perspective the fact that IVF is not a high priority necessitates setting restrictions on the eligibility of applicants. The other factor that must be carefully weighed by each couple is the considerable expense entailed by IVF. At the time of this writing the cost runs from approximately $5000 and upward, a prohibitive sum for many couples. It is difficult, indeed, for a childless couple to evaluate the importance of IVF against its cost, but that cost is enough to make many couples think twice about alternatives to IVF.

The problem of cost raises the question of public support. Leroy Walters, director of the bioethics program of the Kennedy Institute of Ethics in Washington, D.C., has urged that clinical trial testing of IVF should be publicly funded. If it proves successful, then funding should be provided generally. He also states that "a strong equity argument can be mounted for making *in vitro* fertilization and embryo transfer available to all infertile couples who request these services."[11] Such a program could conceivably be financed through private health insurance or incorporated into a public-health plan such as Medicaid. While this is far from being an imminent possibility, it will undoubtedly be proposed if IVF attains sufficient popularity. This is all the more reason for setting careful restrictions on its use, but government support of any kind would likely create a public furor similar to the conflict over abortion.[12]

The argument to allow IVF but to surround it with restrictions does pose problems, for our society may not share a moral consensus on what those restrictions should be.[13] Yet I believe that the public debate raised by this issue could be helpful in clarifying some basic issues concerning our understanding of marriage and the family and what the character of human life is to be. One boundary that appears feasible to me would limit IVF to married couples who desire a child of their own lineage. This would mean that sperm and ova banks would not be allowed, and embryo storage would be limited to facilitating second and third embryo transfers for such couples. The concern here is to resist those inclinations that turn human life in its early stages into a product designed to satisfy a consumer-oriented society. While some would argue that the critical threshold has been crossed already in any utilization of IVF, I believe a significant dividing line based on moral concerns can be drawn on the above basis. At this point it appears likely that satisfying the understandable desire of a relatively few infertile couples to have a child of their own lineage is a sufficient value to bear the attendant risks.

Surrogate Motherhood

Janet Dickey McDowell

Now Sarai, Abram's wife, bore him no children. She had an Egyptian maid whose name was Hagar; and Sarai said to Abram, "Behold now, the Lord has prevented me from bearing children; go in to my maid; it may be that I shall obtain children by her." And Abram hearkened to the voice of Sarai. So, after Abram had dwelt ten years in the land of Canaan, Sarai, Abram's wife, took Hagar the Egyptian, her maid, and gave her to Abram her husband as a wife. And he went in to Hagar, and she conceived (Gen. 16:1-4).

Thus begins the most ancient account of surrogate motherhood within the Judeo-Christian tradition. To those who have followed legal and medical developments in the United States over the last decade, the story of Abram, Sarai, and the surrogate Hagar has a familiar ring: years of marriage with no progeny, despair over the absence of heirs and family life, the fortuitous presence of a woman who might conceive and provide the much-desired child. Contemporary arrangements are, of course, substantially more complicated and differ in many respects from Sarai's simple offering of her slave, but consideration of the increasingly popular practice of surrogate maternity must not neglect the fact that deliberate extramarital conception has had a long history as a means of dealing with female infertility.

The advantages and disadvantages of such a practice and especially its standing within a Christian ethical framework must be assessed just as any other proposed solution to involuntary childlessness is assessed, but surrogate motherhood's relative lack of novelty and its lack of dependence on sophisticated medical support (in contrast to *in vitro* fertilization or embryo transfer, for example) set it apart from most other emerging modes of reproduction. Greater attention must be focused on the potential moral hazards or benefits of surrogate motherhood and less on the medical risks (since they are few). At least four parties must be considered: the potential biological father, his wife (if he is married), the potential biological mother or surrogate, and the proposed child to result from the arrangement. The perspective of each of these individuals will be examined after a description of the contemporary practice of surrogate motherhood and a brief overview of biblical and other theological insights into a Christian view of infertility, procreation, and parenthood.

The Current Practice of Surrogate Motherhood

Most surrogate motherhood arrangements are similar in their basic structure. A woman, designated the surrogate, agrees to conceive a child via artificial insemination and to surrender the child at birth to the man who provided the semen (and to his wife, if he is married). It should be emphasized that the surrogate usually is severing all ties with the child, who is hers genetically. She allows the child's biological father to assume responsibility for the child's upbringing and permits the biological father's wife to adopt her husband's child. All of this is agreed in advance, prior to conception, and may be formalized in a written contract. Ordinarily the surrogate will be compensated for at least her medical expenses.

Beyond this basic framework, surrogate motherhood is a practice almost as diverse as the people who enter into the agreement. Surrogate motherhood is often discussed as though it were one phenomenon when, in reality, there are a great many variations in the way people come to participate in the arrangement, in their motives and reasons for participating, and in their expectations about the future interrelationships among the child, the surrogate, and those who raise the child. Some of these differences in the structure of surrogate motherhood may be morally significant; others may simply be matters of preference or convenience. The most common permutations in the arrangement will be outlined immediately below.[1]

The first variation in the contemporary practice of surrogate motherhood in the United States has to do with the nature of the problem that prevents the man desiring to be a father from conceiving a child in the ordinary way. In the vast majority of reported surrogate arrangements the man is married to a woman who is infertile as a result of any one of several medical conditions.[2] Usually the couple has considered, then rejected, adoption as a means of dealing with their infertility. They may have become discouraged by the scarcity of healthy (especially Caucasian) infants available for adoption, or they may have concluded that they would prefer to raise a child to whom one of them has a genetic connection. They may have difficulty meeting age or other requirements of adoption agencies. Unlike adoption, surrogate motherhood presents the possibility that the husband can make a genetic contribution to the child and that he and his wife can care for the child from a very early point in its life; some couples, with the surrogate's permission, even participate in the birth, and most obtain custody of the child in its first few days of life. Most of the people who seek surrogates fit this pattern and do so because as a couple they are physically incapable of having a child.

However, in a small number of surrogate arrangements there is no medically demonstrated problem preventing normal conception and pregnancy. Instead, the reason for desiring a surrogate is the absence of a wife. Some single men have entered into agreements with surrogates because they want to be fathers but do not want to be husbands. The surrogates can assure them of children of their own without entanglements. Because this reason for entering into the surrogate arrangement is comparatively rare, the majority of this essay will continue to make reference to the male's wife as a party to the agreement. Nevertheless, it should be remembered that not all surrogate structures include an infertile woman; some are created because the man does not wish to have or cannot find a suitable partner for marriage and procreation.

A second striking variation observable in surrogate motherhood arrangements concerns the relationship between the surrogate and the prospective parents. Will the surrogate be a woman already well known by the couple, or will she be a stranger selected from an application form? If she is not already acquainted with the couple, will the three meet prior to and/ or during the pregnancy, or will they always remain anonymous, dealing with one another through an intermediary?

Some of the earliest reported cases of surrogate motherhood involved friends or relatives who had volunteered to be surrogates. Each of these women was apparently motivated by a personal concern for the childless couple known to her, and one would expect that her relationship with the couple and the child continued in some form after the birth.[3]

Other women responded to newspaper advertisements seeking surrogates and agreed to bear a child for people previously unknown to them. Sometimes they met and became close to the couple; in other situations anonymity was preserved. Because artificial insemination is always the means of conception, it is possible to avoid any contact between the surrogate and the couple, but it is not clear whether that is preferable.[4]

Related to the anonymity issue is the heated controversy over payment to surrogates. Surrogates who are related to or close friends with the couple desiring a child rarely if ever seek payment for the service of carrying the child, acting on altruistic or humanitarian grounds, not for any financial gain. Some of the first surrogates responding to advertisements also agreed to the arrangement without compensation beyond medical expenses, citing reasons such as compassion, curiosity, or the desire to experience pregnancy without responsibility for the results. The absence of payment was, in fact, an explicit stipulation in the contracts drawn up for some surrogate arrangements, because to offer or accept any fee beyond medical expenses would have run afoul of laws in many states that prohibit monetary exchanges for the privilege of adoption— laws to prevent a so-called "black market" in babies.[5] However, as the notion of surrogate motherhood was publicized and greater numbers of infertile couples expressed an interest in finding surrogates, it became clear to some involved in the practice that the supply of women who were medically and psychologically suitable to be surrogates and also willing to do so without compensation was quite small; certainly the numbers were not sufficient to meet the perceived demand.

Thus efforts began to legitimate a commercial version of the practice of surrogate motherhood, with fees ranging from $5000 to $20,000 or more. The strategy adopted was to attempt to alter state statutes prohibiting "baby selling" or to establish through the courts that surrogate motherhood did not fall within the proscribed practice (since the child was being surrendered to its natural father, not merely given up for adoption). Some of the earliest attempts failed, but Noel Keane, the lawyer best known for his advocacy of surrogate motherhood, continues to be optimistic that the practice of compensating surrogates will be vindicated and that commercial surrogate motherhood will be found to be compatible with public policy concerns for children's welfare.[6] Some will debate the wisdom of regulating the amount of compensation beyond medical expenses, while others, repulsed by the very notion of any financial remuneration for having a child, continue to argue that no payment should ever be permitted. The legal status of paid surrogates and the couples who provide payments is cloudy at best.

Also related to the anonymity issue is the question of the future relationship among the surrogate, the child, and the infertile couple. Several options are imaginable. The surrogate could establish and maintain a fairly close relationship with the couple and with her child, in which case the child might or might not be informed about the surrogate's biological relationship to him or her. At the other end of the spectrum, the anonymous surrogate might agree to the arrangement through a third party, surrender the child to the couple without coming to know them, and the child might never be told of the unusual circumstances of his conception and birth. Certainly, concealing information about origins was not an uncommon practice until quite recently (when adoptees became more vocal about their rights to access to such material); some may believe it would be in the best interests of both the surrogate and child to sever all relationship between them immediately after birth and perhaps even to withhold the fact that the child is not the natural offspring of both social parents. A middle ground would be making information about the child and his development available to the surrogate at her request and informing the child about the surrogate at some point judged appropriate by the natural father and his wife. Less direct contact would be encouraged than in the first option, especially during the child's early years, but the surrogate birth would not be concealed or denied.

A final difference emerging in the practice of surrogate motherhood has to do with the ''qualifications'' of the surrogate. Descriptions of the current situation suggest that surrogates are screened, with varying degrees of rigor, to rule out women with serious existing health problems or a family history of genetically transmitted disease or defects. But there is no agreement on whether the surrogate should be single or married, whether she should have carried one or more healthy children through a full term pregnancy without complications, or whether there should be age restrictions on applicants. Advertisements have been placed in mass-circulation newspapers, but also in some college newspapers, where they are directed, one assumes, to women 18 to 22 years old. The emotional stability of candidates for surrogate motherhood and their understanding of the physical and emotional consequences of pregnancy may or may not be carefully assessed, depending entirely on the procedure adopted by the persons making the agreement.[7] Individuals who are greatly concerned with the health of the potential child and the welfare of the surrogate may set high standards before embarking on the arrangement; those whose focus is on obtaining a child by whatever means are available may be less scrupulous.

In summary, the designation ''surrogate motherhood'' does not capture the complexity of the many arrangements that carry that label. Careless use of the term may cover up important differences, since it could be referring to a single man hiring an anonymous divorcee to bear his child for $30,000, to an infertile couple arranging with a sister-in-law to carry a child for them, or to college sophomores volunteering to be matched with couples in order to try out pregnancy and pay their tuition. As a first step, an infertile couple contemplating the option of surrogate motherhood would have to clarify the exact sort of arrangement available to them. Only then could they consider the moral implications of the agreement.

A Christian Interpretation of Procreation and Parenthood

Though in the story of Abram, Sarai, and Hagar the Bible provides an ancient account of what might be called surrogate motherhood, the Bible does not deal in any systematic way with this or any other contemporary response to human infertility. The sophisticated scientific understanding of the biological process of reproduction was absent in biblical times, and intervention to relieve childlessness was unheard-of except in the most basic of ways, such as the offering of a substitute for one partner. Nevertheless, the Bible contains substantial guidance regarding the relative importance of procreation and parenthood for those within God's covenant community and indicates a remarkable sensitivity to the psychological and social stresses faced by those who desire children and cannot have them.

Procreation has an honored place in the biblical witness. In the creation narratives of Genesis human beings are created male and female with the potential to ''be fruitful and multiply,'' but only together. From the beginning, both were needed in order to fulfill their promise; human parthenogenesis never seems to have been possible or desirable from God's perspective. Through the companionship and sexual communion of two people committed to one another was to come new life. William Graham Cole argues that ''the Hebrews saw marriage as a cleaving together which created one flesh, perfectly symbolized in the children which were to be expected. They are indeed the blending of two into one in an absolutely indissoluble way."[8] Thus from a biblical standpoint procreation is a joint venture of marriage partners.

Polygamy appears to have been acceptable as a traditional form of social organization and procreation sometimes took place within that context. But procreation was never clearly endorsed in the absence of a stable relationship between the man and the woman, a relationship that was recognized by the community and acknowledged openly by both partners. The difficulties that arose from one of the few apparent exceptions, the aforementioned union of Abram and Sarai's maid, Hagar, were formidable and might stand as a warning of the complications of procreation unsupported by a genuine marital relationship.

Barrenness, particularly as presented in the Old Testament, was a tragedy. Always attributed to the woman (because of the notion of reproduction that prevailed), the failure to have a child foreclosed the most important role available to women in Hebraic society, that of mother, and denied her a substantial component of a woman's worth. Children, especially many children, were indicative of God's blessing and, while the Old Testament did not always explicitly describe barrenness as a sign of God's displeasure, one can imagine that the affected woman would interpret it to be so. The relief of infertility, as with Sarah's conception of Isaac, was the fulfillment of God's promise, a wonderful gift, for then one could fill the earth with descendants, carrying on the family name and preserving its memory.[9]

The importance of parenthood and family to the Old Testament covenant community was further reinforced by practices such as polygamy and the levirate obligation. Lineage was traced through one's father; polygamy permitted a man to produce many children who, though having different mothers, shared a common kinship and loyalty. The levirate obligation was the duty a man owed to a brother who died without offspring. By impregnating the brother's widow, a man could assure that the brother's name would not die with him, since by law the child was considered that of the deceased. Onan, who refused to fulfill this obligation, was punished with death (Gen. 38:1-11). Children were one's primary link to the future, in a sense one's immortality, and so these and other social structures were arranged to ensure such a continuation.

Nevertheless, even with the clear importance attached to the institution of the family and to procreation, at least some elements of the Old Testament temper the focus on children, elements that are picked up and extended in the New Testament. The account of Abraham's near sacrifice of his long-awaited son by Sarah, Isaac, speaks powerfully (if somewhat brutally) of the priority one's commitments should have: obedience to God's command is to take precedence over natural family loyalties and duties, even to the extent that one would be willing to have one's child die.

This theme of ordering one's commitments is echoed and amplified in Jesus' calling of his followers, who must be prepared to leave everything:

> For I have come to set a man against his father, and a daughter against her mother, and a daughter-in-law against her mother-in-law; and a man's foes will be those of his own household. He who loves father or mother more than me is not worthy of me; and he who does not take his cross and follow me is not worthy of me (Matt. 10:35-38).

The demands of the kingdom of God may require the setting aside of traditional bonds in favor of ties created by common dedication to the faith. In one of the most striking challenges to the tightly knit, family-oriented social structure of his day, Jesus is described as responding to a request for a private word with his mother and brothers by exclaiming, "Who is my mother, and who are my brothers?" and indicating that those who serve God have rightful claim to those titles (Matt. 12:46-50). In this and other incidents Jesus appears to be deprecating the traditional Hebrew emphasis on the genetically based family as the crucible for the forging of covenant relationship with God, urging instead an individual commitment the depth of which may strain or even break family solidarity.

Though Jesus urged that the family and one's responsibilities to it be kept in perspective, subordinate—like all lesser loyalties—to one's love of God, he did not advocate its dissolution nor propose any alternative, such as "free love" or communal child care, to a biologically based unit for the procreation and rearing of children. His clear prohibition of divorce and his presence at the wedding at Cana have been seen as buttressing and blessing the monogamous union of a man and a woman as the core of family life—although it is to be a family that turns not inward on itself for ultimate meaning and fulfillment, but outward to find its significance in service to God and God's people. If one's worth and value are not found merely by one's membership in a particular tribe or family linked by blood, neither ought they be bound up with the biological creation of those who will carry on the line.

What conclusions can be drawn from this brief sketch of biblical material? At least two generalizations seem justified, and though they stand in some tension, they do not contradict one another. The first lesson is the great esteem in which the family is to be held, with God's blessing and at his command: parents are to be honored, newborn children to be celebrated as gifts from God, the capacity to procreate through loving intercourse to be cherished, and grief acknowledged when natural procreation is not possible. But the second lesson, equally significant, is that the family is not the only or even the most important dimension of human life; covenant faith with God is. If family demands or concerns jeopardize the relationship with God through Christ and threaten to eclipse the only truly ultimate source of meaning, then the family may have become a substitute for God. Jesus opposed all forms of idolatry, whether idolatries of law, economic status, or family; nothing must take God's place, not even institutions that God has sustained and that the Bible endorses.

How have contemporary moral theologians contributed to the Christian understanding of parenthood and procreation, especially as related to surrogate motherhood? Curiously, much of the current discussion can be divided into two basic camps: a "physicalist" approach that focuses on the importance of the biological family's integrity, and a "spiritualist" approach that emphasizes nonbiological sources of family ties. Both perspectives claim biblical warrant, and both illuminate vital aspects of family life. It is worthwhile exploring these two fundamental understandings of parenthood and examining in some detail their implications for the surrogate-motherhood arrangement.

The following pairs of attitudes demonstrate roughly the physicalist/spiritualist poles with regard to parenthood:

Physicalist	Spiritualist
Parenthood as given	Parenthood as voluntary
Particular children as given	Children as products of series of conscious choices
Families as exclusively biological	Families as solely moral or legal constructions

The items on the left exemplify an admittedly extreme version of the physicalist approach to family life. Whether one is or is not a parent is God's choice (or nature's choice); it is "given" in that sense, not elected, and the absence of children is interpreted as indicative of the divine will. Similarly, whether one's child is male or female, affected by genetic disease or free of it, is not for the parents to choose or control.[10] An external rather than an internal locus of control is perceived by the couple when they contemplate their procreative activity.[11] Taken to its logical conclusion, the physicalist approach to family life would cast doubt on the complete legitimacy of family units that are created without biological connections, perhaps even including adoptive arrangements, for such constructions lack the natural genetic foundation of the family. This may sound bizarre, but surely such an idea underlies the desire some couples continue to harbor to have a genetically related child even after they have adopted, or the commonly articulated reason for seeking surrogate motherhood: so that the child will be "partially ours" or "mine" (when the impetus for the arrangement comes from the fertile potential father).

Despite the partial genetic connection forged by surrogate motherhood, physicalists would unanimously oppose surrogate motherhood. The opposition stems from the importance attached to the physical integrity of the marriage and the implied commitment to procreate with (and only with) the marital partner. To conceive a child by a third party (through artificial insemination by donor, surrogate motherhood, or the newest technology, ovum transfer) is to violate marital fidelity in a fundamental way. Such a practice menaces the biological foundation of the marriage and the family and, as Richard McCormick has argued, "To weaken the biological link is to untie the family at its root and therefore to undermine it."[12]

In contrast, the elements occupying the right half of the spectrum are those engendered by a spiritualist viewpoint. Parenthood is perceived as entirely voluntary (whether through procreation or by legal or social means). It is in essence a moral commitment, not the inevitable result of a physical contribution. When biological reproduction is undertaken, means for controlling the timing of pregnancy and even the sort of child that results (including maneuvers to determine the gender and genetic health of the child) are not merely permissible, but virtually obligatory. To do otherwise would be to surrender human responsibility. Because it discounts or denies the role of biology in creating families, this perspective tends to see the family exclusively as a moral or legal community created by human choice and purpose. Thus the presence or absence of genetic ties among family members is a matter of indifference. Joseph Fletcher asserts:

> The bonds which tie people together are moral, mental, emotional—not biological. Parents, siblings, and kinsfolk are no "closer" to us than our spouses, friends, neighbors, and fellow men in general. What constitutes a genuine relationship is shared caring and concern, not "blood" or genes or genital origin.[13]

There is no reason, according to this view, to prefer that children know and/or be reared by their genetic parents.

The essentially spiritualist position can lead to quite opposite opinions regarding surrogate motherhood. One can see that this perspective could endorse the practice, because the child's absence of a genetic link to its social mother would be inconsequential and the almost purely physical connection between the child and the surrogate would be greatly discounted. There would be little concern over the participation of a third party in procreation, for the focus of moral attention would be on the joint *decision* by the prospective parents to procreate in this way, not on the means needed to achieve their goal. The suggestion that procreation with a woman not his wife compromises the man's marriage vows of fidelity would be rejected as ludicrous, because fidelity is understood also in terms of commitment, not in terms of who receives his sperm.[14]

On the other hand, an individual embracing the spiritualist perspective might oppose surrogate motherhood on the grounds that it was a surrender to a biologically based understanding of parenthood, wrongly encouraging the infertile couple's misperception that a child resulting from surrogate motherhood would be "closer" to them than an adopted child. Surrogate motherhood, and many other means of circumventing infertility, are simply unnecessary; as long as there are some children in the world in need of loving homes, the appropriate response to involuntary childlessness is adoption.[15]

The consensus of moral theologians representing both poles of the debate seems to recommend hesitation about, if not opposition to, surrogate motherhood (though there are exceptions, such as Joseph Fletcher). The reasons cited are disparate and sometimes contradictory, but they provide insights that can be applied to each of the parties involved in the surrogate motherhood agreement. Much of the focus of the discussion of the practice of surrogate motherhood has been on the infertile couple; they are crucial, but the potential for difficulties with the arrangement seems stronger when the surrogate and the potential child are also considered.

Surrogate Motherhood: The Infertile Couple

Would the arguments made by either the physicalists or the spiritualists persuade an infertile couple that surrogate motherhood ought not to be undertaken? Probably not, and not merely because they may be more concerned with solutions to their shared problem than with the niceties of ethical debate. If one looks critically at either perspective, there are sufficient objections to make a middle-ground position appealing. And, *judged solely from the infertile couple's viewpoint,* and from within a more moderate position than either the physicalist or the spiritualist, surrogate motherhood may be morally justifiable—if not commendable.

What is the content of an interpretation of parenthood that stands between the poles of physicalism and spiritualism? It would deny the physicalist's claim that being a parent must be grounded in biology, acknowledging the human capacity to transcend biology and be "mother" or "father" in the most important ways without contributing ova or sperm. But it would also recognize, as the spiritualist's approach does not, the abiding links forged by biology. Thus it would be sympathetic to the man's desire to procreate, to engender a child genetically connected to him without disparaging that man's wife's capacity to nurture and love a child with whom she has no such connection. "Unequal" relationships to children are not uncommon; stepparents have needed to cope with such an imbalance and have done so, one imagines, with varying degrees of success. As long as both potential legal and social parents are willing to make an unqualified commitment to the child, it does not seem that the child's origins in a surrogate arrangement would necessarily jeopardize their relationship to the child.

More serious objections stem from the effects of the surrogate situation on the relationship between the man and his infertile wife and the distortion of the full meaning of procreation that the surrogate arrangement entails. Both biblical material and the commentary of some contemporary moral theologians argue that the begetting of a child ought to be the result of loving communion between its parents.[16] The conjunction of the joys of sexuality and the potential reproductive functions is not held to be incidental. Deep communication and rich pleasure are conjoined with the giving of new life. There are, of course, many instances in which children are conceived without love between sexual partners, without permanent commitment, without an intention to be responsible for the child, but these are tragic, often sinful situations—not normative ones. Surrogate motherhood requires that the husband procreate (however anonymously) with a woman with whom he has no relationship even vaguely approximating a marital one.[17] It is true that his behavior can be called "adulterous" only by a very strict interpretation of that term and that couples involved in the surrogate arrangement have not themselves perceived it as any betrayal of marital fidelity; nevertheless, it is surely procreation outside the marriage, and as such it falls short of the Christian norm for procreation. The end—a child specifically conceived for the couple and sharing the man's genetic constitution in part—does not ordinarily seem sufficiently serious to warrant such a major distortion of procreation. However, one can imagine circumstances in which this breach of the procreational norm might be justified—cases where there are very few or no adoptable children available or where the couple fails to meet some arbitrary criterion to qualify for adoption—and so, seen from the infertile couple's perspective, surrogate motherhood might sometimes be considered.[18]

Surrogate Motherhood: The Surrogate

From the viewpoint of the surrogate, it is hard to imagine how one could justify the surrogate-motherhood arrangement. This may seem surprising, since it has been the willingness of women to volunteer to serve as surrogates that has popularized the practice in recent years. But in light of Christian norms and values, there seem to be few if any factors that would support a woman's decision to become a surrogate, and there are many that should discourage her. This appears to be the case whether the surrogate knows the infertile couple or not, is married or single, is compensated handsomely or carries the child without remuneration. Some of these variations may be more problematic, but in any of the possible permutations, human procreation is reduced to the status of a service for hire (or for donation), and the surrogate is encouraged to engender an attitude of distance and alienation from her own child and her body. Neither of these outcomes is compatible with a Christian notion of giving life.

Surrogates have been quoted as saying that they agreed to conceive a child and subsequently give it up for a number of reasons: curiosity; to assuage guilt over an earlier abortion; because pregnancy and birth had been or were expected to be personally rewarding experiences; or, most frequently, out of compassion for childless couples. Whether these reasons are interpreted as selfish or altruistic, both biblical and contemporary resources indicate that by themselves they are not appropriate reasons for undertaking procreation. There is no context of loving commitment to the child's father, a basic prerequisite; and unlike the husband within the infertile marriage, the surrogate has no intention to care for the child she deliberately conceives. The absence of these crucial elements reduces human procreation to the mere biological production of babies; whether the surrogate is paid or not, she has misunderstood the essential character of procreation and so degraded it.

Of the cited reasons, compassion would seem to be the least objectionable, the reason a Christian woman might be moved to become a surrogate. Compassion is commended biblically, and there can be great sorrow associated with an infertile couple's plight, sorrow that may be alleviated only by a child. However, it must be recognized that there are limits even on behavior stemming from sympathy. If an individual offered to shoot himself in the head to provide a heart or other vital organ to someone in need, the individual's action would be discouraged, no matter how sincere the desire to help.[19] A person who robbed a bank to help the poor or, in a less dramatic vein, drained her child's education fund in order to support a worthy charity would also be vulnerable to criticism, especially because the person could be seen as sacrificing someone else's interests in order to demonstrate compassion. Surrogate motherhood may be somewhat analogous to the latter example, particularly if one concedes that the child may have some interest in knowing and being reared by its genetic mother. Therefore it is not unreasonable to argue that surrogate motherhood is compassion gone awry, sympathy that steps beyond the bounds of appropriate behavior. The deliberate conception of a child outside of wedlock is not a matter of indifference, and being motivated by concern for unhappy people cannot compensate for the moral deficits inherent in the action.

In defending their decisions to become surrogates, some women describe themselves as "providing the gift of life"— an action which on its surface also appears commendable. But a Christian understanding of procreation does not view children as entities to be created in order to be bestowed on others, as though they were handmade sweaters or cookies. Participation in their creation necessarily entails a responsibility for their welfare, a commitment to try to meet their physical, emotional, and spiritual needs; the surrogate has absolutely no intention of carrying out that responsibility. There are certainly other contexts in which one or both of the biological parents may be unwilling or unable to behave responsibly, in which case others may fulfill the parental role, but, again, these are not normative situations. Moreover, the premeditated character of the surrogate's decision to forfeit the parental relationship makes her choice especially repugnant.

In conclusion, it seems difficult to imagine circumstances that would warrant a Christian woman's choice to be a surrogate. Though her motives may be praiseworthy and her concern for childless couples genuine, she fails to appreciate the full value and responsibility of procreation. Surrogates who conceive primarily for financial reasons have strayed even farther from the norm, and so perhaps are more subject to censure, but all surrogates seem confused about the appropriate use of the reproductive capacity.

Surrogate Motherhood: The Potential Child

Implied in much of the foregoing discussion is a concern for the child who might be conceived as a result of a surrogate agreement. Describing the best interests of a potential child is a difficult task, since any flaws in the situation into which he is born must be balanced against the "problem" of never being conceived at all. This is frequently pointed out by advocates of surrogate motherhood—that without the cooperation of the infertile couple and the surrogate the particular child would never exist. But no one has ever argued that all potential children ought to exist, and Christians regularly try to consider a potential child's interests when making judgments about family size or the prudence of conception when the probability of genetic disease is high. Assuming that there is some value in being conceived and born, are there reasons that one might not wish to encourage conceiving and bearing children in a surrogate arrangement—for the child's sake? There may be.

The primary pitfall from the child's perspective is a confused or nonexistent relationship with his mother. If the individual contracting with the surrogate is single, the child would most likely be raised without a mother, since the supposed purpose of the surrogate arrangement for a single male is the potential of raising a biologically related child without making commitments to the child's mother. Single persons have been permitted to adopt children in many states and often seem capable of providing loving, stable homes. But the surrogate situation differs by being premeditated: there was never an intention that the child have a substantial relationship with two parents. This seems less than fair to a child and may show a lack of concern for the child's best interests, a concern that perhaps ought to overrule a single person's desire for a biological child.

The more common surrogate arrangement, in which the infertile wife adopts the child, provides the child with two parents, but the question of the child's connection to its biological mother still needs to be resolved. It is possible that the couple might not inform the child of his or her unusual origins, allowing the child to believe the social mother had given him or her birth. In addition to being a violation of the Christian commitment to truth, such deception could be very difficult to maintain. Should the child learn the truth from others, the child's trust in those who have done the rearing could be greatly undermined.

If the infertile couple chose instead to be candid with the child, the issues of trust and truthfulness might not arise, but other problems almost certainly would. If the couple acknowledged the child's surrogate birth but severed all ties with the surrogate, the child would be cut off from an important source of medical information, not to mention the less tangible contributions to personal identity that come from knowing biological kin. Whether the child met and came to know the surrogate or not, the child might feel divided loyalties between mothers, or a sense of rejection, since the biological mother never wanted the child herself but always planned to give the child away. Payment to the surrogate could complicate the child's response: what would it mean to know your mother had been paid to conceive and carry you to birth? These may not be insurmountable difficulties, but anyone considering surrogate motherhood surely ought to be aware that the child will be faced with many of the same kinds of questions and doubts that adoptees voice—and the surrogate child would have the additional burden of knowing that the separation from his or her natural mother was the result of choices freely made by the adults around the child, not the result of circumstances they could not control.

Surrogate Motherhood: The Whole Picture

Taken as a whole, does surrogate motherhood appear to be an arrangement Christians would condemn, condone, or applaud? The picture is a mixed one, but the majority of the evidence leans against surrogate motherhood. Wholesale condemnation may not be appropriate, but Christian perceptions of the significance of procreation and its place within the marital relationship are not compatible with the basic premise of surrogate motherhood: that one could deliberately conceive and bear a child with no commitment either to the child or to its father. From the perspective of the infertile couple, surrogate motherhood may appear to be a tempting solution to a heart-wrenching problem, and the child that would result would experience the awesome gift of life. But do these benefits really outweigh or justify the distortion of procreation that makes them possible? Ultimately this is a judgment that might best be left to individual conscience, but it should be a conscience informed by the Christian community and the Bible. Parenthood is affirmed as good, but only when it is kept in perspective. There is a grave danger faced by all parents but heightened by the desperation felt by infertile couples—the danger that a child may replace God, as revealed through Jesus Christ, as their center of value and meaning. Children are wonderful gifts entrusted by God, but they are not gifts to be sought at any price. For most people the costs of creating a child through surrogate motherhood—costs to the integrity of the marriage, to the surrogate's self-understanding, and perhaps to the child—are simply too high.

4

Genetic Manipulation

—James H. Burtness—

Genetic manipulation has to do with rearranging, adding, or deleting genetic material for the purpose of bringing about desired changes in living things. There are varieties of procedures and goals, and varieties of opinion on the propriety of some or all of these procedures and goals, particularly as they relate directly to human beings. It is the purpose of this essay to introduce the reader to this phenomenon, to supply some basic information about it, and to suggest some lines along which attitudes and positions may be developed, specifically by adherents of the Christian faith. An underlying assumption is that Christian faith can, ought to, and often does influence ethical reflection, but that it rarely yields direct or uncomplicated responses to ethical questions.[1]

The church in which the degree of certainty about its moral judgments exceeds the degree of certainty about its faith commitments has already shifted its center from proclamation and confession to moral instruction, and that moral instruction is often less helpful and even more dangerous than ''secular'' ethical reflection because of the power of the divine authority on which it often too quickly calls to support its judgments. The reader, therefore, who is looking for "the Christian answer" to this problem will be disappointed in this essay. It is hoped that the reader looking for some material further to stimulate reflection will find the essay helpful.

After posing the fundamental question, the essay will comment on some voices of caution, including a recent statement about genetic manipulation that was signed by many Christian leaders in the United States. Following this, an attempt will be made to give a historical perspective to the present situation, to look at some ethical issues, and to point to some Christian resources for reflecting on these issues.

The Question

Science usually begins with observation and moves toward manipulation. First there is the quest for new knowledge, then the question of how to use that knowledge. Research leads to application. The attempt to understand the power within nature is followed by the attempt to exercise power over nature. It is highly unlikely that humankind will ever be content to sit and observe. It is difficult to imagine, for instance, that anyone would suggest that the world population would have been better served by simply observing the spread of smallpox, rather than by intervening with procedures which have eliminated it. Few people, if any, would like to do away with the electric light bulb or the telephone. Most people expect that science will not only acquire information, but that the information will be used to solve problems and to benefit life.

This expectation, however, is both limited and complex. It seems obvious to most people that not everything that can be done ought to be done. That point need not be labored. Power over nature can be destructive as well as creative. It can hinder life as well as assist it. Most people would like to retain the electric light bulb, but rid the earth of nuclear weapons. Some things that seem at first to be only helpful—the use of certain pesticides and fertilizers for example—are found later also to be harmful. Even medications prescribed for specific illnesses often have known side effects, and occasionally those side effects have been discovered only after they have done considerable damage to a segment of the population. The aesthetic delights of basic science bring along in their wake the ethical quandaries of applied science.

The question is thus not whether to manipulate nature. Everyone who mows a lawn or takes an aspirin manipulates nature. And everyone agrees that there are times and ways in which nature ought not to be manipulated, although they do not agree on what those times and ways are. The question is, therefore, how and when to do it, within what limits, under what circumstances, in accordance with what rules, toward what ends. A given procedure ought to be regulated, or prohibited, not because nature ought never to be manipulated or because humans ought never to "play God," but because the particular procedure under consideration ought for specific reasons to be done only under certain conditions, or perhaps ought not to be done at all. Only since the early 1970s has genetic manipulation in the laboratory become a live ethical issue, because only since then has it become possible, due to the development of a procedure known as recombinant DNA research. Use of this procedure is today a commonplace event. But there are people who counsel great caution, particularly about its use in connection with human genetic material.

Voices of Caution

Caution is too mild a term for the opinion of some critics. There are those who regard the new manipulation of genetic material as comparable to the manipulation of the atomic nucleus. Four decades ago Hiroshima and Nagasaki signaled the coming terror of the age of nuclear weapons. There are some biologists who fear a similar pattern of events resulting from what they consider to be misuse of their discipline. Included in this group is Liebe F. Cavalieri, professor of biochemistry at the Graduate School of Medical Sciences, Cornell University, and long-time associate of the Sloan-Kettering Institute for Cancer Research. He himself did pioneering work in the molecular biology of DNA, the carrier of the genetic code in every living thing. Cavalieri writes:

> The discoveries that energy can be released from the atomic nucleus and that DNA, the material of the cell nucleus, is the genetic stuff of life are without parallel in human experience. These twin scientific feats, one at the core of matter, the other at the core of life, demand a new consciousness if human life on this planet is to continue.
>
> We have mismanaged the applications of the first discovery. Now, as the second is about to be exploited, we must not permit the biosphere, surpassing as it does our understanding, to become an experimental subject. There is only one Earth, one earthly biosphere, and we are a part of it. There is no margin for error.[2]

Cavalieri was one of the very few scientists who signed a document, authored by Jeremy Rifkin, that was released to the press on June 8, 1983. There were 63 signatories, most of them church leaders. They represented a broad spectrum, from Jerry Falwell of the Moral Majority and Pat Robertson of the 700 Club to an impressive list of mainline Protestant and Roman Catholic bishops. Also signing were a few well-known theologians and ethicists. Among them were J. Robert Nelson of Boston University and Richard McCormick, professor of Christian ethics at the Center for Bioethics, associated with the

Kennedy Institute in Washington, D.C. After a number of "whereas" clauses, the resolution reads: "Resolved, that efforts to engineer specific genetic traits into the germline of the human species should not be attempted." The resolution is worth mentioning only because Rifkin was able to persuade so many Christian leaders to sign it, and because of the attention given to it by the press. Typical was the full-page story in *Time* magazine, entitled "Scientists Must Not Play God," introduced with the sentence "Seldom, if ever, in the U.S. has there been so ecumenical a chorus of concern."[3]

The release of the Rifkin resolution did not coincide with any new discovery in molecular biology or any new development in gene splicing. Any application of the technique to human body cells is, in fact, thought by many people working in the field to be only a distant possibility, and there is no indication that insertion of new genetic material into the human germline is a current threat. (In the first case—genetic manipulation of the somatic or body cells—any change brought about would die with the individual. In the second case—genetic manipulation of the germline—such change would continue into successive generations.) That with which the press release did coincide was the publication of a book by Rifkin, entitled *Algeny*.[4]

By training or profession Rifkin is neither theologian nor scientist. He is director of his own Foundation on Economic Trends, a Washington-based political-action organization. It took him a full year to get the support needed to orchestrate this media event, and he had to compromise his own position considerably in the process.[5] Even at that, many of the people who signed the resolution had second thoughts once they saw the way in which it was used. Twenty-four Roman Catholic bishops signed the document, yet the National Conference of Catholic Bishops has made it clear that it does not endorse the resolution. The Reverend Avery Post, president of the United Church of Christ and a signer of the Rifkin resolution, said later: "I believe this society is capable of dealing rationally with such an indisputably beneficial therapy, if the bioethical forums are in place."[6] Cal Thomas, an aide to Jerry Falwell, told reporters: "Dr. Falwell sought only to issue a call for comprehensive national discussions. . . . He would support those changes which would be life-enhancing."[7] Richard McCormick of the Kennedy Institute told reporters that he is not certain of his position, but "signed not to prohibit research forever, but to try to encourage public debate."[8] Many science writers responded to the public excitement over the Rifkin resolution with amazement. *Discover* editorialized: "The clergy may possibly be excused for being taken in by this kind of pseudoscientific blather. . . . [but] scientists who are taken in by his nonsense ought to be ashamed of themselves."[9] There does seem to be among many religious people an almost innate antipathy toward the scientific enterprise, which explains Rifkin's decision to enlist supporters from the religious community and to attach to his resolution a so-called "theological statement." Nevertheless, there are also voices of caution from the scientific community. The word from Professor Cavalieri has already been cited. Also signing the Rifkin resolution were Nobel laureate George Wald, professor of biology at Harvard University, professor of biology Ethan Signer (MIT), professor of biology Ruth Hubbard (Harvard), and professor of chemistry Kurt Mislow (Princeton).

Not even the most enthusiastic supporters of genetic manipulation think there are no risks, but they advise caution, not prohibition. Alexander Capron, professor of law, ethics, and public policy at Georgetown University, served for three years as executive director of the President's Commission for the Study of Ethical Problems in Medicine and Biomedical and Behavioral Research. The final report of the commission came in 1983. After an eloquent description of scientific risks and ethical concerns, Capron writes:

> At this point in the development of genetic engineering no reasons have been found for abandoning the entire enterprise—indeed, it would probably be naive to assume that it could be. To expect humanity to turn its back on what may be one of the greatest technological revolutions may itself betray a failure to recognize the limits of individual and social self-restraint.
>
> Assuming that research will continue somewhere, it seems more prudent to encourage its development and control under the sophisticated and responsive regulatory arrangements of this country, subject to the scrutiny of a free press and within the general framework of democratic institutions.[10]

In a similar vein, Jonathan D. Moreno, assistant professor of philosophy at George Washington University, writes in the *Hastings Center Report:*

> In the end, the germline issue may serve mainly to draw public attention to the problems raised by rapid developments in genetic engineering generally. There is reason to doubt that regulation of lucrative and widely desired genetic procedures could be enforced over the long run. Human egg cells are not the sort of commodity that is easily restricted and experiments in this country and abroad would be immensely difficult to police. Rather, a new commission would create a context for education and the exchange of views, one that might provide what Clifford Grobstein called for in his testimony before the Gore subcommittee: an "accommodative wisdom to guide the new age of genetic and developmental intervention that clearly lies ahead."[11]

When one encounters the careful work of the president's commission and of people who are actually engaged in the research, one is struck by the sobriety of their reflection, the modesty of their claims, the civility of their argumentation.

Christians who respond positively to those traits are apt to be embarrassed by pronouncements that appear to be arrogant or heavy-handed or careless. It is important to have some historical perspective to see that the present situation is one link in what has been and probably will be a long chain of events. The question is whether this one link is qualitatively different from all others or so different in magnitude that the difference in degree constitutes a difference in kind. There are, as is often the case, capable people on each side of that question.

Historical Perspective

New forms of plant and animal (including human) life have been evolving since those modes of life first appeared on this planet. Adaptations have been made from the beginning by living things to various environments. Some adaptations entered the germline and have been passed on from one generation to another. Not all genetic evolution has been strictly involuntary. Some changes have taken place by design, so that there is a sense in which selective breeding of stock animals and the development of hybrid grains constitute a kind of primitive manipulation of genetic material. Desired changes have been brought about by purposeful manipulation of reproduction. Nor has this selective breeding been restricted to plants and animals. It is perhaps offensive to those who embrace strictly romantic notions about love and marriage, but a great many people in various cultural settings have attempted to arrange "good marriages" for themselves or their children, and in doing so have paid some attention to factors of family health and intelligence. What had been going on for many centuries in an informal way began to move into a more scientific phase a little more than a hundred years ago. The Augustinian monk Gregor Mendel began in 1854 to keep records on smooth and wrinkled peas, and formulated his conclusions 12 years later. These

"Mendelian laws" for simple dominant and recessive genetic traits are still the basis of genetic science, although many modifications have taken place over the years.[12]

A century after Mendel began his work, James Watson and Francis Crick in 1953 published their initial paper on the structure of the DNA molecule. In 1962 they received the Nobel Prize for their work. About 10 years later, the new knowledge moved into the stage of application. There were many steps along the way, and it is impossible to fix an exact date, but about 1973 the technology was in place to manipulate genetic material in the laboratory. The process had moved from observation to manipulation, from information about the power within nature to methods by which to exercise power over nature. The procedure is called "recombinant DNA research" or, more popularly, "gene splicing."

The DNA molecule is an extremely long chain of strictly ordered subunits, a length of several hundred to several thousand of which is called a gene. Genes are contained in chromosomes, made up primarily of DNA and some associated proteins. All sexually reproducing organisms have pairs of chromosomes in all body cells (humans have 23 chromosome pairs), one chromosome of each pair inherited from the father and one from the mother. When an egg and a sperm combine, each carrying a single set of chromosomes, those chromosomes also combine into pairs, and the genes function according to the now familiar laws for dominance and recessiveness. Every cell of a given organism carries the same chromosomes, and thus the same genetic information is copied exactly every time a cell divides—that is, almost every time. Once in a few hundred thousand times there is a mistake, a mutation, in the copying of the genetic information. In almost every case the mutant cell does not survive. However, in an incredibly small number of instances, the mistake happens to be a "good" one, and the cell is "improved," made stronger, more able to survive in its environment; therefore it continues to live and to reproduce. According to current evolutionary theory, there is good reason to believe that all life present on earth, from human beings to bacteria, is the product of several billion years of mutation, recombination, and selection.

Human beings have never been willing to allow this evolution to take place in a purely haphazard fashion. From the beginnings of civilization, farmers have been intervening in the course of evolution by producing hybrid grains, and stock breeders have been domesticating animals that live longer or work harder or run faster. The new datum in our time is the development by molecular biologists of procedures that make it possible to control this recombining process (so that it is not simply "random"), and to increase almost immeasurably the speed by which it takes place.

The technology involved is somewhat analogous to the development of the computer. Electrical impulses have been occurring in the human brain for as long as human beings have been on the scene. As an extension of the human brain, the computer enables that same process to go on in a more controlled and exceedingly more rapid manner. Recombinant DNA technology, then, does not involve doing something that has never before been done. It does make possible a quantum jump in the degree to which humankind can take control of the evolutionary process, including the evolution of human beings.

Recombinant DNA research has thus far been done primarily on bacteria, one-celled organisms smaller than animal or plant cells and simpler in structure, yet capable of complex chemical activity. The bacterium which has been the chief vector, or vehicle, for DNA research is *Escherichia coli* (*E. coli*), genetically and biochemically the most completely analyzed organism on earth, having been grown and studied in laboratories for more than 50 years. It is also extremely common, living in the intestines of many animals, including humans.

By using restriction enzymes, it is possible to open up a plasmid (a self-replicating circular piece of DNA) and then match it up with a piece of DNA from any source that has been acted on by the same enzyme. These two pieces are cemented together by the action of another enzyme, called a DNA ligase, and the new recombinant molecule, or plasmid, is inserted into an *E. coli* bacterium. When the cell divides, it reproduces the recombinant plasmid in each new cell. This technology thus makes it possible to produce not only the recombinant DNA, but also unlimited quantities of new organisms created in the laboratory.

Almost immediately after the technology became operative, a series of events moved toward the establishing of regulatory devices for monitoring the research. The Gordon Conference on nucleic acids in the summer of 1973 was followed by an open letter to *Science* magazine, which was in turn followed by the establishment of the Recombinant DNA Molecular Program Advisory Committee in October 1974 by the National Institutes of Health. In 1975 there was an international conference of scientists at the Asilomar Conference Center in California at which a temporary moratorium was called by the scientists on certain kinds of DNA research. A great deal of publicity was given to the Asilomar Conference, and some people responded in panic. The city council in Cambridge, Massachusetts, went to battle against Harvard and MIT, attempting to prohibit the research at those institutions. Boards of regents of major universities, and also state legislatures, sought to regulate the procedures. Bills were introduced into Congress. Out of this flurry of excitement guidelines were established for both physical and biological containment of the research. For a few years scientists worked in an atmosphere of relative calm.

Two major events occurred in 1980. In June the United States Supreme Court ruled in a 5-4 decision that new forms of life could be patented. The decision was the culmination of an eight-year legal battle between General Electric and the United States government, a battle the government finally lost. The court decided that a new human-made variation of the common bacterium *Pseudomonas* could be brought under the patent laws, originally written in 1793 by Thomas Jefferson. Jefferson wanted to be sure that "ingenuity should receive a liberal encouragement" and that "any new and useful art, machine, manufacture or composition of matter" was patentable and thus legally protected from theft.[13] The new bacterium was developed in the General Electric laboratories at Schenectady, New York, by microbiologist Ananda M. Chakrabarty. The bacterium has a huge appetite for oil, and turns the oil it eats into protein and carbon dioxide. Although it has never been done, in theory these bacteria could be manufactured, kept freeze-dried until needed, then spread over straw on an oil spill in the ocean. They would ingest the oil, multiplying as they gorge themselves, breaking down the oil into protein and carbon dioxide. When the oil is gone, according to inventor Chakrabarty, the bacteria would simply starve to death, having nothing more to eat to keep them alive. Although commercial genetic engineering firms were in place prior to the Supreme Court decision, it is obvious that industrial gene splicing was given new incentive by the court.

The other event in 1980 was the beginning of work by the President's Commission for the Study of Ethical Problems in Medicine and Biomedical and Behavioral Research. The mandate of this commission was a broad one, but it included work on genetic manipulation. This commission was appointed by President Carter, partially in response to a letter from representatives of Protestant, Catholic, and Jewish groups alarmed by what they considered to be a movement "into a new era of fundamental danger triggered by the rapid growth of genetic engineering."[14] That commission delivered its report on March 31, 1983. Also in 1983 came the Gore resolution for a new presidential commission,[15] and the Rifkin letter and resolution already mentioned above, accompanied by the publication of Rifkin's book *Algeny*. At the time of the writing of this essay, 1984 is upon us, together with all the fears of Orwell's *1984* and Huxley's *Brave New World*. The developments in genetic manipulation are indeed awesome. Whether one reacts in fear or in hope depends as much on one's basic perspective on life as it does on the procedures themselves. Yet some knowledge of procedures is essential if one is to achieve an informed opinion, because it is the procedures themselves out of which the ethical issues arise.

Some Ethical Issues

The title of this essay, and the main term around which the discussion has moved thus far, is "Genetic Manipulation." There is a variety of terminology used to designate these procedures, however, and the meanings of various terms overlap. There is considerable lack of precision, for instance, in distinguishing uses of the terms "genetic manipulation" and "genetic engineering." In sorting out some issues, it is necessary to select terms and assign meanings to them, even if it has to be done somewhat arbitrarily.

The term "genetic surgery" is sometimes used. A more specific term for this procedure might be "gene transfer." It is, however, sufficiently analogous to surgery so that the terms "corrective gene transfer" and "elective gene transfer" can be used as code words for the same procedure used for different purposes. If the use of terms is restricted to direct manipulation of human genetic material, neither is currently practiced, nor is the practice of either anticipated in the near future. Yet a great deal of discussion is already taking place because of the probability that both will eventually be possible. In each case, some form of recombinant DNA procedure would be employed. "Corrective gene transfer" refers to the correction of a genetic defect. "Elective gene transfer" refers to the enhancing of an individual's genetic endowment. The distinction is an important one. It is similar to distinctions such as "genetic treatment" and "genetic enhancement," or "negative eugenics" and "positive eugenics," or "corrective surgery" and "elective surgery," or "preserving life" and "prolonging life," or "avoiding harm" and "doing good." The distinction is important because some people argue for "corrective gene transfer" and against "elective gene transfer." However, although the distinction is important, is it not necessarily clear.

If it is decided that both of the above terms be used to describe genetic manipulation of somatic (body) cells, then "germline manipulation" can be used for the same technology applied to germ cells (sperm or ova). The distinction here is that genetic changes in somatic cells die with the individual, but genetic changes in germ cells are passed on to that person's progeny. Here the distinction is both important and clear. There are people who argue for the use of DNA technology on human body cells, whether one considers the procedure as "corrective" or "elective," but argue against the use of the same procedure on human germ cells. There are others, however, who argue for correcting "defects" in both body and germ cells, but against using the same technology to "enhance" life, whether in body or germ cells. And there are those who oppose all uses of DNA technology on human cells, and those who oppose all such opposition. People who struggle with these issues cannot be easily categorized, however, even when the complexity of options is recognized. There are many who bring a degree of sophistication and subtlety to these questions that defies casual labeling and necessitates careful engagement.

If, however, "corrective gene transfer," "elective gene transfer," and "germline manipulation" are used as code words for the direct use of DNA technology on human cells, it is important to recognize that there is a very large area in which the same technology functions for the benefit (according to proponents) of human life, but only indirectly. No direct uses are currently operative. Some uses indirectly beneficial (or thought to be so) are in place, and a great many more are anticipated. Again, there is a variety of opinion. There are those who oppose all forms of recombinant DNA research of whatever kind for whatever ends, although one can say with confidence that the number of such people has decreased dramatically since the technology was first introduced about 10 years ago. On the other hand, there are those who are enthusiastic about the use of the technology to benefit humankind indirectly but who oppose direct use of the same technology on human cells. And there are those who see no sharp line between direct and indirect benefits— and risks. To round out our somewhat arbitrary designation of terms and definitions, let us use "biotechnology" to refer to uses of recombinant DNA technology that seek to benefit human life without actually working on human genetic materials. The scope of actual and anticipated benefits is overwhelming.

The Supreme Court decision on the oil-eating bacterium developed by General Electric has already been mentioned. Advanced Genetic Sciences of Greenwich, Connecticut, has developed a way of adding the bacterium *Pseudomonas* to the water used in snow-making machines to increase their productivity, particularly at warmer temperatures. Benefits that seem frivolous to some are obviously important to others. Insulin and interferon can probably be produced commercially by biological factories, making these materials vastly more accessible than they have ever been. There is an entire new science of protein manufacture, including the design of new hormones, antibodies, and enzymes. This is not genetic manipulation of human cells as such, but the industrial manufacture of new organisms, which in turn produce hormones, antibodies, and enzymes used by the human body. It thus has the potential of altering human life perhaps as greatly as does human gene transfer.

The use of a growth-hormone gene, manufactured by biotechnology, to produce "supermouse" was much publicized. Most of us think mice are already large enough, and the thought of new generations of giant mice is enough to cause almost anyone to say no to the entire enterprise. It looks a bit different when one realizes that this laboratory animal will not reproduce itself, and that the growth-hormone gene developed through these experiments could benefit the 10,000 American children who now suffer from one type of dwarfism. At the present time the hormone comes from the pituitary glands of cadavers, and it takes from 50 to 80 cadavers to provide a single year's dose for a single child.[16]

There is now a simple way of triggering disease-fighting responses by the body's immune system. By copying short sections of proteins—parts of disease viruses—researchers have succeeded in creating experimental artificial vaccines for hepatitis, diphtheria, and other diseases. "We can make an antibody to any reasonable protein we wish," says Richard A. Lerner, chairman of the Department of Molecular Biology at Scripps Clinic in California.[17]

The same process applies to the manufacture of enzymes. Enzymes play a catalytic role, "promoting one or more particular chemical reactions, singling them out for innumerable reactive possibilities in the bewildering complex environment of a living cell and doing so at rates far outstripping most other chemical reactions."[18]

The Holy Grail would be to synthesize artificial catalysts, based on what we know about enzymes. . . and tailor-make catalysts for a variety of industrial purposes. Imagine mining gold or other precious elements from ordinary seawater—where concentrations are minuscule but total amounts are vast—by merely adding a solution of artificial enzymes. Imagine biochips and whole computers made of artificial proteins, as powerful as today's supercomputers but too tiny to be seen by the naked eye. Imagine proteins that would stimulate humans to regenerate damaged organ tissue, grow a third set of teeth, or regrow severed nerve fibers, mimicking embryonic development.[19]

The protein engineers dream of massive benefits to human beings brought about by the manufacture of proteins by biotechnology. It is still in the future, but nobody knows how soon these things could be commonplace.

Although work has been done on plants for some years, progress is extremely difficult and slow. One reason is that the genetics of plants is far more complicated than is the genetics of either mammals or bacteria. String beans, for instance, have 10 times the DNA that human beings have. In bacteria a single gene usually determines a single trait. In plants, however, the ability to extract, or "fix" nitrogen from the air seems to be determined by a complex set of at least 17 genes. Yet it is theoretically possible so to engineer the DNA of plants that no fertilizer would be necessary. Nitrogen could be obtained from the air. It may even be possible to engineer plants that will ward off pests, making pesticides unnecessary, or plants that could live virtually without water, or that could use the sun more effectively in the photosynthesis process, or could grow in salty soil. Creating new plants is one problem. Propagating them is another. Cloning works at the present time in only a very few plants—carrots, petunias, and tobacco. But important cereal grains and legumes, like soybeans or peanuts, do not respond at all well to cloning.[20]

What can be said about ethical issues arising out of such a vast and complex set of experimental procedures and industrial technologies, particularly when word about some new break-through appears in the press almost every week? How is it possible to handle with any expertise and clarity the entire grid of possibilities of opinion having to do with distinguishable procedures we have chosen to label "corrective gene transfer," "elective gene transfer," "germline manipulation," and "bio-technology"? There are specific issues associated with specific procedures. For instance, one would have to speculate about what would happen if General Electric's oil-eating bacterium did not die when the oil spill was consumed, and one would have to do that aware of the actual properties of the bacterium and the probability projections of such a thing actually taking place.

Such thinking presupposes the validity of risk/benefit anal-ysis. A large and general issue is whether such analysis is even appropriate. People who think that "tampering with nature" or "playing God" is inherently wrong are not going to bother calculating risks and benefits of a specific procedure. Those also who have made a large decision that the probable risks of DNA technology are not warranted by any possible benefits are also not going to bother calculating risks and benefits of specific procedures. A scan of the literature, however, makes it clear that most people who reflect on these issues do consider that risk/benefit analysis is essential to ethical reflection. One finds articles speaking about "the blessing and the curse,"[21] or "the promise and the peril,"[22] or "the prospects and the hazards,"[23] or "the thrills and the chills."[24] The question re-mains whether such calculating is appropriate when doing eth-ical reflection in a Christian context, or whether Christian faith must drive a person to an unqualified affirmation or unqualified rejection of these procedures. The answer to that question depends in part on the resources to which one appeals in the Christian Scripture and tradition.

Christian Resources for Ethical Reflection[25]

To the question, "What does the church have to do with the genetic manipulation debate?" some Christians answer "Nothing." Christianity is, they say, a religion for personal salvation or for the preservation of eternal values. Others maintain that there is a simple and direct line from Christian commitment to a given position on such matters. They say, opposing genetic manipulation, that we ought not to "play God" or, favoring it, that God had given human beings "dominion" over the creation.

Contrary to both of these extremes, the position taken here is that Christianity provides, in addition to the word of the gospel, some materials from which certain conclusions can be drawn, however tentatively, about the nature of reality and of history, that theology involves the clarification of the church's proclamation but also the attempt to delineate the church's stance toward the world and toward every new event and idea.

There is no simple and direct move from the Bible to a position regarding genetic manipulation. There are, however, implications of biblical faith that may help to inform possible responses to the ethical issues raised by the debate. Let us consider five such implications.

1. The Christian outlook on reality and history cannot be adequately summed up as either optimism or pessimism but, if a choice is to be made, the church must stand with the optimists.

To say that Christians are going to be either optimists or pessimists is much too simple. The prophetic motif of salvation in and through historical process and the apocalyptic motif of salvation crashing in from outside of history are intertwined in the biblical documents, and each motif needs to be qualified by the other. There have always been Teilhard-style "optimists" and Ellul-style "pessimists" in the church, and the church needs both. But the Christian faith has a lean toward optimism. G. K. Chesterton, who happened to agree, described the pessimist as a cosmic antipatriot, and the optimist as one who has a supernatural loyalty to things. He said that any act of cosmic reform must be preceded by an act of cosmic allegiance.

Christians who believe in the creation of all things by a benevolent (and beneficent) God, in his enfleshment in Jesus of Nazareth, and in the eschatological resurrection of the body have a persistent loyalty to matter and to things, which invites an act of cosmic allegiance. The Christian can never be a naive optimist, because Christianity insists that demonic realities and possibilities be taken seriously. There will, however, be a steady tilt toward expecting good results from new discoveries about the nature of things.

In the biblical documents, the prophetic motif dominates the apocalyptic, which implies that hope characterizes the Christian stance toward life. *Hope* is a better word than *optimism*, for it excludes naivete, invites participation, and encourages the thoughtful directing of those processes over which we have some control.

Hope also assumes that there will never be absolute security about anything, that "conditions of uncertainty" will always prevail, that this is, in Norbert Wiener's words, a "probabilistic world." That view does not mean that no decisions can be made with confidence, nor does it mean that one decision is as good as another. It does mean that relativities always have to be taken into consideration, that data always have to be weighed, that we are always dealing not with what will necessarily happen but with what will probably happen, that decisions always carry some risks. The Christian ought never to be frozen into inaction because of the presence of risks or the absence of complete data, although a given action may be specifically rejected because the risks are too great in the light of the data available. Doubt ought always to be qualified by hope rather than by despair.

The church has a great stake in the future and anticipates it with positive expectations. If a new procedure, such as genetic manipulation, appears to be full of promise, the tendency ought to be toward investigating its possibilities.

2. Because the outlook of the church is characteristically full of hope, its expectations of the future ought to, and often do, feed back into the making of current decisions.

There is a long tradition in ethics, focusing in the work of G. E. Moore, that insists that it is impossible to derive an "ought" from an "is." (The philosophical analog of that tradition is Lessing's famous dictum that it is impossible to derive eternal truths from historical facts.) Because Protestants have tended to be idealists philosophically and Kantians ethically, they have often assumed that values and facts, or morality and data, have very little to do with one another. Albrecht Ritschl, in fact, stated that quite bluntly.

It is difficult to see, however, how it is possible to take the theological *eschaton* (the last things, the kingdom of God, the new heaven and the new earth) seriously without also taking the ethical *telos* (goal) seriously. Teleology, the ethical methodology that calls an action good if it produces good results,

though more at home in the Roman Catholic than in the Protestant tradition, cannot be entirely excluded from any decision-
making process that claims to be Christian. Moving with hope-
ful confidence into the future on the basis of the data of God's
past and present action in our history is simply what Christianity is about. Thus there can be no a priori reason for ruling
out cost/benefit analysis as a device for making decisions, even
those having to do with something as potentially destructive
as genetic manipulation.

Furthermore, there seems to be specifically Christian wisdom at work in talk about the "ethics of long-range responsibility," or in John Rawls' insistence that the notion of justice
be expanded to include justice to future generations. The Christian has a peculiar stake in the long run—one which the Hindu,
for instance, with an essentially spiritual outlook on life and
a cyclical view of history, can never be expected to represent.
If it is true that the sins of the fathers (and mothers) will be
visited upon the third and the fourth generations, surely it is
also true that the responsible and wise and loving acts of the
fathers (and mothers) will be visited upon the third and the
fourth generations.

If we worship a God who is from the beginning to the end,
who is both Alpha and Omega, then we ought to be able to
walk into the future confident that the creating and redeeming
God is truly with us, now and to the end of the age. So we
can dare to calculate consequences, to analyze costs and benefits, precisely because we believe that this is what God does
as he works with his world, moving it ever closer to the final
consummation of his purpose for all things and all people.

C. P. Snow once suggested that scientists have the future
in their bones, while humanists tend to look back longingly to
a distant golden age. One of the ironies of history is that, given
a choice between siding with humanists or with scientists, most

Christians tend to choose the former. Of course it is finally a false alternative, but the tendency persists. If the church's theology were informed more by biblical expectations of a redeemed creation and less by general religious longings for ecstatic experience and timeless truth, Christians would find themselves at the very least congenial toward those who, with a passionate "loyalty to things" and a "cosmic act of allegiance," struggle to unpack the secrets of life on this planet and to work with this life toward a new day.

3. The Christian who operates from a stance of hopefulness, believing that God is working through human history and through the history of nature, will be inclined to place the burden of proof on those who oppose a given type of scientific research.

Christians know very well that it is impossible to do anything without making mistakes. The whole creation is not only imperfect; it is out of joint. There can be no such thing as zero-risk research. In fact, the entire history of science could be told as the story of attempts to devise methods by which mistakes can be "good" ones—that is, mistakes that are reversible and from which we can learn something. The specific problem in assessing genetic manipulation is the fear that a mistake will be made that is not reversible, that cannot be corrected, and that will bring misery to us all.

If the potential benefits of genetic manipulation were negligible, there would be no problem in deciding not to do it. Given, however, the benefits projected and the possibility of regulation, the burden of proof must be on those who think the procedures should be stopped.

The whole cluster of arguments against "playing God" and "tampering with nature" must, in any case, be rejected summarily. We are constantly creating things in our own image, but that may be quite appropriate if we really believe that we are created in God's image. Although the creature must be sharply distinguished from the Creator, that does not rule out a relation between the two. The creative itch was placed in the creature by the Creator, and so long as we remain human we shall be working with him, and he with us, to preserve and to redeem things and situations and people. The question is never whether we will alter nature, but rather how we do it, and to what purpose.

The apostle Paul asks the church at Rome: "If God is for us, who is against us?" (Rom. 8:31). He says to the church at Corinth: "For all things are yours, . . . and you are Christ's; and Christ is God's" (1 Cor. 3:21-23). The Christian, more than anyone, expects good things to happen. Einstein, perhaps unconsciously, was gathering up some profoundly biblical insights when he said: "God is subtle but he is not malicious." Not everything that can be done should be done; potential costs will often outweigh potential benefits. But in a world in which good things are expected to happen, in which hope rather than fear is the dominant motif, the burden of proof will lie on those who decide in a given instance that a specific laboratory procedure—in this case genetic manipulation—should not be done.

4. Since Christian faith is tied to the passing on of information rather than to the repetition of an inspiration, the church will always have a special interest in the acquisition, interpretation, and dissemination of knowledge.

Paul writes to the church in Corinth that he is only passing on to it what has been passed on to him, namely, that Jesus Christ died, that he was raised, and that he appeared. Although he had as great a "spiritual experience" as any person in history, Paul rarely mentions it. He sticks to the "facts" about Jesus. Those are interpreted facts, of course; there are no such things as uninterpreted facts. But they are nevertheless facts, data, information. When it has been true to itself and its mission, the church has promoted literacy, encouraged learning, established universities, and founded libraries. Its darkest hours have been those times when it has lost touch with its origins and turned against those who sought or found new information about the world or about human life.

B. F. Skinner is correct when he insists that there be no areas of human life excluded from investigation, even the areas labeled "freedom" and "dignity." And the same goes for anything labeled "mystery." The Christian who knows that God made all things "in, through, and for" Christ ought never to fear any new information about anything. The church thus has an enormous stake in the preservation of academic freedom, and not just the right of professors to think up great ideas—in fact, not particularly for that at all. Instead, its interest is in the research that is constantly at work to find out as much as possible about what makes things tick, whether organic or inorganic, living or nonliving.

And Christians know that thinking and acting are distinguishable, but inseparable. From the very beginning of Genesis, word and deed are partners in doing. So, speaking, no less than acting, is potentially dangerous as well as potentially beneficial. Freedom can never be absolute and will always have to be subject to some kind of regulation in any specific setting. Genetic manipulation can be encouraged by the church as one more way to acquire information about and to work with our world, but it must also be subject to some form of regulation, as must every other human enterprise.

5. *Because of its confidence in the redemptive possibilities of human activity, the church will tend to think that regulation is possible; because of its awareness of the demonic potential of human activity, it will insist that regulation is necessary.*

Reinhold Niebuhr said the same thing about democracy. Augustine, in his struggle against Manicheanism, on the one hand, and Pelagianism, on the other, said it long before Niebuhr. It also holds true for the church's attitude toward genetic manipulation. Any attempt to stop the work entirely (in other countries as well as in the United States) would not only be unrealistic; it would be contrary to basic commitments of the Christian faith about God and the world. But to encourage the conducting of the work with no controls is to court disaster at the hands of overly zealous (and ambitious) individuals who may well be more concerned about satisfying curiosity or achieving fame than about promoting the common good.

There is no reasonable alternative to regulation; hence the church, if it acts wisely, will attempt to be in conversation not only with those who set up regulatory procedures, but also with those who carry them out. Any procedure is going to require constant monitoring and frequent alteration. We have been busy at that task with nuclear energy for a quarter of a century, and there is no reason to believe that the regulation of genetic manipulation will be any easier, or any less necessary.

Where does that leave the church? The answer is, as "a piece of the world redeemed by Christ," as Bonhoeffer was fond of saying. The church has no right to expect to be heard automatically, as though its authority is somehow self-evident. However, because church people know and proclaim him who is Lord of all, the church will—if it is true to its Lord and to itself—speak with concern and passion about those things that have been learned regarding this creation, and about those things that are yet to be learned, about those things that have been done and those things yet to be done. And, from time to time, the world will recognize in its speech an authentic and helpful word.

Genetic Screening and Counseling

James M. Childs Jr.

A mother: I don't think we should ever do anything to prevent the conception or the birth of a defective child like our Suzy. I believe she is part of God's plan. We never knew what love was all about until she came into this world. In fact, if it weren't for her and others like her, maybe you scientists wouldn't be motivated to discover all of these cures which benefit everyone.

Augenstein: Let me ask you two questions. Do you really believe that you and your husband can ever justify learning to love, if your child has to pay the price of a lifetime of extreme suffering? And can you believe in a God who would give you your wonderful brain and then not expect you to use it to spare Suzy her continual, aimless misery—if you could? That is not the God I believe in! In fact, I don't need suffering little Suzies to spur me on. Rather I need to be sure that people like you will use new information responsibly and humanely. Otherwise we scientists might as well stop right now.[1]

Many readers will doubtless recognize this dialog as coming from the late Leroy Augenstein's once popular book, *Come,*

Let Us Play God. The dialog opens Augenstein's chapter on genetic defects and neatly poses the challenge that pervades his whole book: ". . . We can never be God. However, God has given us dominion over the earth. Since man's increasing knowledge now forces him to make decisions of life and death that cannot be sidestepped, come let us make them together—humbly and prayerfully, but above all responsibly."[2] As we investigate the manifold ethical questions in the field of genetic screening and counseling, the issue that Augenstein so graphically raised is still with us.

Theological Context

Knowledge is a marvelous thing, but knowledge imposes responsibility. As Augenstein correctly sensed, this notion of responsible use of knowledge is, for people of biblical faith, rooted in the doctrine of our creation in the image of God. As the image of God, we are persons in intimate relationship with God, uniquely endowed with the capacity to know, the freedom to choose, and the corollary responsibility to choose well how we use that which we know in the loving care and control of ourselves and our environment. To *own* this responsibility is to recognize our moral constitution as human beings. To *exercise* this responsibility in ethical reflection and decision making is to encounter another truth about ourselves: we are sinners who inhabit an imperfect world which has been "groaning in travail" with us.[3] That is to say, our struggles with moral reasoning and the agonizing dilemmas we encounter in our decision making frequently lay bare, to those who are sensitive, the ambiguity of our motives, our often perverse priorities, and some of our frightening capacities to be selfish and unfeeling under the cloak of doing what is good for all concerned. Even when our motives and intentions appear to be at their noblest, ethical dilemmas are often so intransigent as to leave us with no feeling of moral certitude after we have done our best.

This is not to say that Christian ethics and its application to real-life problems is to be equated with the *law* in the theological sense that the Reformers used the term *law,* to refer to the accusation of God's Word against our sinful estrangement from God and one another. However, in and through the process of applying ethical principles to perplexing questions of decision, the truth of what the law reveals about the human predicament is often evident as we struggle with our motives and recognize in the radical ambiguity of some of our decisions the tragic character of our world, whose full redemption is not yet consummated. In the pain of moral choice we appreciate ever anew our desperate need for the new life that is ours in Christ Jesus.

To embrace the new life in Christ is to be able to craft our ethical principles, analyze our situations, and make our decisions free from the perils of self-deception and self-justification, complacency or despair. We are freed by God's acceptance of us in the Christ to be realistic, self-critical, and bold. In short, new life in Christ empowers us to proceed in humility and confidence.

The focus of this chapter is the ethical issues that arise in genetic screening and counseling. I hope to explain, analyze, and provide guidance. However, all our discussion is framed by these briefly stated theological perspectives on ourselves and on God's merciful activity in our lives. Bioethics is but one instance of applied ethics; applied ethics is but one instance of our encounter with God and ourselves.

Understanding Genetic Defects

Before we can begin to deal with genetic screening and counseling, a brief description of the knowledge about genetic defects should be useful in providing a hint of the magnitude and severity of genetic disease. Scientists have now identified more than 3000 different genetic disorders. Recent figures indicate that one or more of these defects appear in more than 200,000 infants out of a total of three million born each year in the United States. Two to three percent of that total show major genetic or congenital disease. An article in *Newsweek* further estimates that genetic disorders account for 30% of the children and 10% of the adults in our hospitals.[4] It is this significant genetic burden that has given so much impetus to the development of genetic screening and counseling in our time.

Genetic disease is transmitted from one generation to the next by one of four different types of inheritance.

1. The first of these is *inheritance due to a dominant genetic trait possessed by one of the parents.* Unless there has been a new mutation, the parent possessing the trait will suffer from the same disorder he or she passes on to the child. With dominant traits there is a 50% chance that offspring will manifest the disease. If a child is born with a dominant defect due to a new mutation in either the egg or sperm cell at the time of conception (a situation in which neither parent has the disease), there is little likelihood of another occurrence in subsequent children. In a case in which one of the parents does suffer a dominant disorder but their child is normal, the child will not transmit the disease to his or her offspring.

Well-known dominant genetic disorders include *achondroplasia* (a form of dwarfism), *glaucoma, hypercholesterolemia* (high cholesterol levels with a propensity to heart disease), *polydactyly* (possessing extra fingers or toes), *neurofibromatosis* (tumors in the skin along the course of the peripheral nerves), *Ehler-Danlos syndrome* (excessively soft joints subject to frequent dislocation, loose and fragile skin, easy bruising and calcified cysts),[5] and *Huntington's chorea* (progressive degeneration of the central nervous system). Huntington's chorea is particularly insidious, because it usually develops in adult life, often in the middle years, giving ample opportunity for passing on this terrible and fatal disease to a new generation without even realizing the risk. In general, dominant traits are either mild or appear later in life, but many cause physical and emotional suffering, and some are lethal. Reproduction is not usually affected.

2. The second type of inheritance is that of *recessive genetic defects.* In the case of recessive genetic traits, both parents (who are usually normal or unaffected) must have the defective gene. When this occurs, there is a one in four chance that their child will be afflicted with the disorder. If the child does not manifest the disease, the chances are 50-50 that he or she will be a carrier of the trait, who must then be concerned about whether or not his or her mate will also be a carrier. Recessive genetic defects most often cause serious and frequently fatal birth defects.

Four of the better known recessive defects illustrate their severity. *Sickle-cell anemia* is a blood disorder primarily affecting blacks. Red blood cells in the victim take on a "sickle" shape and clog the flow of blood. As a result there is severe pain and damage to the tissues throughout the body. Few with sickle-cell anemia live past 40, and many die in childhood. *Tay-Sachs disease,* most common among those of Eastern European Jewish ancestry (Ashkenazi), is an invariably fatal condition involving brain deterioration. As the disease progresses, the child suffers loss of muscle control, blindness, deafness, paralysis, retardation, and finally death, by age five in most cases. *Cystic fibrosis* is the most significant genetic disease affecting the general white population of the United States, striking one in every 2500 births per year.[6] In cystic fibrosis there is a mucous buildup that interferes with both digestion and breathing. Treatments have improved life expectancy but only half live to age 20.[7] Our final example is the *PKU (phenylketonuria) syndrome,* a deficiency of an essential liver enzyme, which leads to mental retardation. Currently, most states require screening of all newborns for PKU. Those with a positive test result can be placed on a special diet to forestall the effects of the deficiency. This practice of metabolic screening is itself controversial. Though it is outside the scope of our discussion to deal with that controversy, screening or testing for the purpose of diagnosis and therapy is part of the general discussion of genetic screening.

3. A third form of inheritance is called *X-linked or sex-linked.* The following quotation describes the recessive variety of this inheritance succinctly.

> X-linked inheritance (sometimes called sex-linked)—normal females have two X-chromosomes. Normal males have one X and one Y. Usually, a clinically normal mother carries a faulty gene on one of her X-chromosomes. In such a case, each son has a 50/50 risk of inheriting that gene and manifesting the disorder. Each daughter has an equal chance of being a carrier like her mother, usually unaffected by the disease, but capable of transmitting it to her sons. No male to male transmission of X-linked disorders can occur. That is, a father cannot pass the disorder on to his son.[8]

Males affected with a recessive X-linked disorder will pass the defective gene to all their daughters, who will then be carriers but not diseased. In the case of dominant disorders an affected father will pass the disease on to all his daughters but not his sons. Two well-known X-linked diseases are *hemophilia* and *muscular dystrophy.* According to the March of Dimes there are 205 confirmed or suspected diseases in this category.[9]

4. Finally, a sizable group of genetic disorders is due to *polygenic or multifactoral inheritance.* These diseases are the result of many genes interacting with one another and some-

times with environmental factors. Since the pattern of transmission in polygenic diseases is far from clear, "Persons suffering from these disorders are probably often unaware of any hereditary basis of their disease and fail to obtain genetic counseling."[10] One of the best-known genetic defects thought to be polygenic is *spina bifida*. The total number of defects attributable to multifactoral inheritance is unknown.

In addition to these four forms of genetic inheritance, other birth defects are due to chromosomal abnormalities. Chromosomal diseases result when chromosomes are broken or rearranged. They also occur when there are extra or missing chromosomes. Best known of the chromosomal anomalies is *Down's syndrome*, which we used to refer to as mongolism, characterized by mental retardation and a variety of physical abnormalities. The probability of occurrence or recurrence is strongly related to the age of the mother, the risk increasing with age.

As our knowledge of genetic defects and our ability to detect carriers of defective traits increases, the possibility for prediction and prevention is enhanced. Thus, the promise and urgency of genetic screening and counseling grows with our knowledge—and so do the ethical challenges. Is the public interest such that screening should be mandatory? Are mandatory programs an invasion of privacy and a threat to freedom of choice in reproduction? Is it right to risk a pregnancy when there is a threat of genetic disease? How much, if any, risk is acceptable? How does the relative severity of the disease at risk affect our moral responsibility in procreation? These and other questions come rushing in.

Screening for Detection: Promise and Problems

Certain recessive disorders are peculiar to specific populations. The overwhelming number of sickle-cell anemia cases, for example, occur in the black population. Given this situation and our ability to run tests that will determine who is a carrier of the trait, it has become possible, and many think desirable, to target this population for mass screening programs. The desired goal of such public programs is to reduce the incidence of these diseases by alerting potential parents, who are detected as carriers, of the risks they encounter in their offspring if their mate is also a carrier. In addition, those who learn that they are not carriers are given peace of mind. The benefits of large-scale screening programs to those at risk and to the general public health seem obvious and the rationale for the programs clear. However, a number of problems and questions have arisen.

One of the first difficulties encountered in the sickle-cell screening programs was the threat of stigmatization. Public screening programs are often susceptible to being misunderstood. In some of the sickle-cell programs some people, even physicians, got the impression that being the carrier of a trait is itself a disease. The psychological impact is severe enough when one believes oneself to be flawed or ill, but it is even worse when others believe it too and discriminate against you. Thus, for example, carriers found their insurance premiums raised and their employment opportunities limited.[11] Beyond these unwarranted occurrences, a number of well-intentioned laws passed by various states shortly after the sickle-cell test became available in 1970 further contributed to the problem of stigmatization. These state laws mandated periodic screening. Since the only real benefit to the black population was a warning against reproduction between two known carriers, members of the black community voiced the objection that the thrust of these laws was to reduce the growth of the minority black population. Indeed, the Kentucky law did explicitly restrict the mandatory screening to those ''of the Negro race,'' raising the question of an unconstitutional denial of basic rights.[12]

It is obvious, then, that respect for the equal dignity of all persons requires great care in setting up mass screening programs for specific populations. Community participation and education are necessary to head off stigmatization. Furthermore, programs need to be voluntary rather than mandatory in order to reduce the chances of public discrimination. In fact, many of the states which enacted mandatory laws out of good intentions have replaced them with voluntary ones out of sensitivity to the problem of stigmatization.[13]

In 1970 a blood test was developed to detect carrier status for Tay-Sachs disease. As soon after this as was technically feasible, plans were begun for screening of the Jewish population in the Baltimore–Washington, D.C., area. This program was considered a model effort, everything that the worst instances of the sickle-cell programs were not. Fourteen months of cooperation between professional religious and community leaders went into preparing and educating the community in order to avert the dangers of misinformation and stigmatization. The program was voluntary; the response was gratifying. Similar follow-up programs resulted in more than 100,000 Jews being voluntarily screened in the United States by 1975.[14] However, while it is common to hold up the history of Tay-Sachs screening as a prime example of an effective and ethically responsible program, not all agree with that assessment.

Madeleine J. Goodman and Lenn E. Goodman have criticized Tay-Sachs mass screening programs. Beyond questioning the relative effectiveness of mass screening versus private testing by physicians with their patients, the Goodmans believe that the educational programs utilized have had a damaging psychological effect on the Jewish population. Specifically, they claim that anxiety is the motivational tool used to encourage participation, with the effect that confidence in Jewish marriages and cultural identity is eroded, and genuine, rational free choice is compromised. They fear stigmatization in terms of the self-image, not only of those detected as carriers, but of Jews as a group: "For the group there is the external problem of apparent scientific confirmation of age-old prejudices about racial debility, clannishness, and the like; and the internal problem of the discouragement of marriage and reproduction between Ashkenazi Jews." [15] In the final analysis, the Goodmans contend, stigmatization of target populations seems inevitable because such populations are singled out for special action when, in fact, genetic defects are found throughout the human community; there is no pure breeding stock. [16] Regardless of how one evaluates the Goodman's arguments over against those of the proponents of screening, who cite its benefits and cost-effectiveness, their concerns are not easily dismissed. Psychological manipulation of target populations and the stigmatization that can result are instances of dehumanization. They remind us of a primary concern in all bioethical reflection: our use of scientific knowledge should be geared to the whole person, not merely to his or her genes or symptoms or diagnosis. That is, people must first and foremost be treated as people, not as "cases" or "problems."

Another dimension of concern for the whole person is respect for individual privacy. Obviously, some of the problems mentioned in connection with sickle-cell programs were due to a lack of adequate confidentiality. Safeguards are particularly urgent in mass screening programs, because they are usually done outside the normal doctor-patient relationship. While professional ethics mandates confidentiality in that relationship, it may not be uniformly operative among all involved in

public screening programs. In view of this, one research group
has concluded:

> We favor policies of informing only the person to be screened
> or, with his permission, a designated physician or medical
> facility, of having records kept in code, of prohibiting storage
> of non-coded information in data banks where telephone com-
> puter access is possible and of limiting private and public access
> only to anonymous data to be used for statistical purposes.[17]

That there may be limits to confidentiality is a matter to consider in the next section, but, generally, the principle stands.

Other considerations beside those mentioned are also important to insure that screening programs are humane and responsible. Concern for the well-being of each individual
requires that screening be accompanied by opportunities to
follow up with counseling so that individuals with positive tests
will have the guidance they need to make informed choices.
Similarly, genuinely free and informed consent to participate
in a screening program can be complete only if persons know
what, if any, therapies exist for themselves or their offspring,
should results be positive.[18] Naturally, every effort must be
made to insure safety and accuracy. Promptness in reporting
results is also not without its importance as a way of caring
for people who are doubtless already quite anxious.[19]

Ethically responsible genetic screening programs will be voluntary, informed, and sensitive to the needs of the whole person. Therefore, while recognizing the benefits of screening for
the prevention of suffering, ethicists tend to be cautious about
their advocacy of such programs and concerned about an over-
zealous application of genetic knowledge and screening techniques to unprepared populations in unprepared communities.
There is a particular fear that we may move toward mandatory
screening programs that will not only constitute an invasion of

privacy in the most elemental areas of choosing a mate and reproducing but will also tempt us to legislate "normalcy" *de facto* and slacken our resolve to accept and care for the "abnormal." Ethicist Paul Ramsey speaks for many in this regard:

> While I approve in principle of screening with the prevention of conception in view, it nevertheless should be said that since there are other values in life besides the biological perfection of the individual, some severe qualification may have to be introduced. In the face of mounting possibilities for mass screening, we need to keep in mind that coercion is still an evil. Also, in the face of mounting genetic information, there may indeed be a "right not to know," if all of life's spontaneities are not to be toned down to the impersonal level of the laboratory or all of us learn to smell disease everywhere. For genetics in the future, as for multiphasic health testing, at some point we may have to judge the human costs and benefits of medicine as a whole in comparison with other human needs. Concerning, in particular, future applications of genetic knowledge, we may need to appraise the human costs to follow from a widely held elevation in our expectations of human "normality," with its concomitant lessening of our care for "abnormals" or acceptance of them.[20]

Still, while ethicists may feel their cautions are justified, some in the medical and research fields see their counsel as confused and troublesome, an impediment to progress. Advocates of more aggressive programs see mandatory genetic screening through new public health policy as the most effective way to reduce human suffering, ease the social burden, and promote the human genetic good for future generations.[21] Thus, the debate goes on between the rights of individuals not to know and not to be coerced in reproduction decisions, on the one hand, and the interests of society as a whole, on the other hand. The issue is further complicated by the danger of health professionals confusing good intentions with an ambitious desire to control human destiny through scientific conquest. However, regardless of the relative merits of arguments over public-policy options and the benefits and liabilities of mass screening programs, there remains in the middle of it all the abiding reality of individuals struggling with the dilemmas of decision making. Even though genetic screening is now done primarily on an individual basis, the ethical issues associated with public policy questions should not be allowed to recede from view.

Counseling for Prevention: New Decisions and Old Concerns

New genetic knowledge has brought about new decision-making situations that never existed before. Facing new decisions is the lot of both the genetic counselor and the persons who seek counseling. Yet for all the new decisions, the concerns are as old as ethics itself: respect for the freedom and dignity of each individual, confidentiality (its necessity and limits), the obligation to do no harm, and respect for the sanctity of human life, as well as its quality.

The genetic counselor is a relatively new breed of professional who is still in the process of establishing basic principles for ethically responsible practice. At this writing there are only 275 genetic counselors certified by the American Board of Medical Genetics. Indeed, that board was only begun in 1980 and to date has offered the certification examination only once.[22] At the same time, there are many uncertified genetic counselors who may be functioning with only a master's degree. This situation itself has raised concern about uniformity of professional ethics along with uniformity of qualifications. Some argue that only those trained at the doctoral level, preferably the M.D., working in a medical setting, can provide *relative* assurances of reliable and comprehensive diagnoses in the sort of atmosphere of respect and confidentiality that has been long-standing and deeply ingrained in the medical profession.

Be that as it may, there are a number of concerns about the comportment of genetic counseling that deserve at least brief notice. One such concern has already been encountered in connection with screening, that of confidentiality. The moral requirement of keeping all information about a patient in strictest confidence hardly needs arguing, but does this requirement have its limits in genetic counseling? The issue of limits is raised in a situation in which persons are diagnosed by the counselor as carriers of a genetic defect but wish to keep that information from children or close relatives; perhaps they are hiding the facts about an institutionalized or afflicted child. The counselor recognizes the importance of this hidden genetic knowledge to relatives who could be carriers as well. Must the counselor nonetheless keep confidentiality? Some say they have no choice morally or legally. However, there are legal precedents of immunity from breach of confidentiality for physicians who are dealing with patients afflicted with contagious diseases. There are also precedents in case law for ''conditional'' immunity, allowing the physician to disclose confidences for the protection of a few people, even though the larger society is not affected. These precedents suggest that the legal tradition does not consider confidentiality an absolute when other lives are threatened. At least some commentators favor extending those precedents to the area of genetic counseling.[23]

To break confidentiality is to betray a trust or break a promise. For Christian ethicists who work with rules at all, promise keeping has always been a clear case of a norm that embodies love's concern and respect for the neighbor. However, the norm that commands us to do no harm and to guard the well-being of the neighbor is of equal standing with our obligation to promise keeping. In the kind of situation we are discussing, the counselor finds himself or herself in a conflict between these norms. To me, more is at stake in guarding the well-being of family members who need to know than in keeping the promise of confidentiality. In different situations the decision may appear less clear. Nonetheless, however one decides, there is no avoiding the anxiety involved in the resolution of conflicting claims. We are put in mind once more of the burden of responsibility, and the need for the courage that comes with the freedom of grace.

An additional ethical concern having to do with the design and direction of genetic counseling is the degree of directiveness the counselor should exert. Does genetic counseling simply provide information or also advice? For many, if not most, genetic counselors, the ideal is to be nondirective, leaving counselees to make their own decisions about having children in the face of stated genetic risks. The ethical principle being protected in this view is respect for the *autonomy* of persons. The evil to avoid is paternalistic manipulation of the client. It is generally recognized that good ethics maximizes the possibilities of autonomy and that paternalism compromises our respect for the dignity and responsibility that must be accorded each individual.[24]

However, good ethics also interprets its norms in terms of the reality of circumstances. The reality of genetic counseling situations is that even the most intelligent counselee probably cannot arrive at an understanding and a decision without the benefit of dialog, particularly with the sensitive counselor whose knowledge and experience can be very valuable. Autonomy can often best be promoted through the kind of sharing that enables an individual to think through the choices and considerations he or she needs to be aware of to make a responsible decision.[25] The dialog that involves the discussion of values can well be the servant of autonomy. In fact, the well-informed pastor can be a key person in the process of decision making. Not only can he or she assist with basic understanding of the facts, help deal with feelings of guilt, anger, and questions of why this has happened, but also with a basic understanding of the ethical choices that are consistent with the person's faith. Some genetic counselors welcome the pastor to the team. Even more of this involvement by pastors should be encouraged.[26]

Our discussion of autonomy brings us finally to the responsibilities of the counselee, the parents or prospective parents who have come for genetic counseling. Usually these are persons who have already had one child who suffers from a birth defect. Others are concerned about some disorder in the family history that they suspect may have been genetic in origin. Finally, members of certain populations, such as those at high risk for sickle-cell anemia or Tay-Sachs disease, may come after participation in a screening program or in lieu of such participation. As things now stand, these are the persons who have the final say as to how we use our genetic knowledge.

The first decision such potential parents must make is whether or not to avail themselves of the genetic information that testing and counseling can provide. The temptation to remain ignorant and let nature take its course is a strong one in view of the difficulty of the decisions that come with being informed. Some may even prefer to leave matters "in God's hands." To be sure, all our lives are in God's hands, but God has also given us the responsibility to take care for much of our lives and our world. In general, I assert that we have an obligation to seek the knowledge we need if we have reason to suspect problems with our genetic heritage. Such knowledge can enable us to prevent pregnancies that could lead to the birth of a child who will suffer or maybe even die a painful death. A desire to avoid facing this knowledge is understandable but possibly self-centered and certainly shortsighted. Even the apparently heroic willingness to accept whatever comes along and to care for a child with severe birth defects can be an expression of underlying pride in our own self-reliance or our own convictions. Some may choose not to know for some reason of conscience. It is not the business of ethics to be judgmental and condemning of persons. It is the responsibility of ethics, however, to make judgments about the choices persons confront.

Of course, this general admonition to seek knowledge for responsible decision making might be qualified by the features of particular situations. In some cases the ethics of knowing are more complex. A true case study helps to make the point. A woman came to her obstetrician, concerned that her sister had just given birth to a boy who had a classic case of hemophilia. She was informed that because hemophilia is an X-linked or sex-linked disorder, if she herself were a carrier there would be a 50% chance that any male children she had would have the disease and a 50% chance that any of her female offspring would also be carriers. Her own probability of being a carrier was one in two as well. Her doctor informed her that there is a test to determine whether she is a carrier, but it is only 80-95% effective. If she were to become pregnant, the use of amniocentesis (a procedure for drawing fluid from the amniotic sac and analyzing fetal cells suspended in the fluid) could tell her if she were carrying a male child. However, if she were carrying a male and chose to abort, there would be a 50% chance of aborting a normal child. To make the choice even more difficult, she also learned that only slightly more than half of hemophiliacs have the most severe kind of bleeding problems, and those who do can be helped by new and effective, though very costly, treatments. Should she feel obliged to take the step of being tested for her own carrier status?[27]

The question of abortion complicates this and other cases of genetic counseling where genetic diseases can be detected *in utero* through amniocentesis. The question of abortion decisions after prenatal diagnosis is one that belongs to another chapter. However, the ethics of knowing remains our concern here. This case is not that unusual. Sisela Bok, a philosopher working in bioethics, asserts that the woman in question is obligated to seek the carrier test. Should the test be positive, she favors the alternative of foregoing pregnancy. Dr. Bok regards this course of action as the only responsible reaction to the threat of suffering and of harm to the well-being of the family. By contrast, Mark Lappé, a well-known writer and researcher in biological sciences and bioethics, believes that the woman and her husband might justifiably refuse the carrier test and go forward with a pregnancy, provided they are genuinely ready for the worst. In this view the morality of not knowing is built on the overriding moral decision to take the risks and shoulder the burdens no matter what, without being confused or troubled by test results.[28]

In this hemophilia case the question of whether or not to know all the facts possible has many of the same dynamics of decision as those faced by parents who have already decided to seek counseling and the maximum possible knowledge. Our brief survey of genetic diseases at the beginning of the chapter provides a good sampling of the sort of information one may receive from the counselor. Parents are presented with odds and, from case to case, with the possibility of a birth defect with varying degrees of severity and varying degrees of susceptibility to treatment. The threat of hemophilia may look very different from the terror of Tay-Sachs. Another example is in order. There is a dominant genetic trait that causes a cancerous condition of the eye called retinoblastoma. This was once invariably fatal in childhood but now can be treated through removal of the cancerous eye. Those surviving such a procedure can go on to live otherwise normal lives. But should they reproduce and risk a 50% chance of passing on this genetic trait and submitting affected offspring to the same radical surgery? Should they do so realizing that the continuance of this pattern will gradually increase the incidence of the disease?[29]

Space does not permit us consideration of a sufficient number of cases to map the full extent of the ethical terrain. We shall have to be content with articulating a general norm to consider in all decisions in which significant genetic disorders are possible should parents go ahead with a pregnancy. The severity of many of the genetic disorders that we cataloged earlier and others that could also have been described should give affected and carrier parents pause in asserting the right to reproduce, whether the risk is one in two, one in four, or even considerably less. The obligation to do no harm and to respect the sanctity of life through respect for its quality as well as its propagation strikes one as the overriding ethical consideration. It is a norm that is constant in most ethical systems and one that is manifestly consistent with the ethics of Christian love. The obligation to do no harm counsels against risking pregnancy under the threat of severe genetic disease. To be sure, the decision not to have children and to deal with the abiding feelings of frustration and inadequacy is a grievous prospect but one that is upheld in its reflection of the self-sacrificing character of love.

In the discussion of screening we noted the moral counsel of many ethicists to refrain from mandatory screening or legal constraints against reproduction because of ramifications for the invasion of privacy and for the development of adverse public attitudes toward those with birth defects. However, the protection of personal freedoms at the level of public policy does not mean that individuals facing the risk of genetically diseased offspring should feel totally free from moral constraint. Similarly, the importance of nurturing humane attitudes of care and acceptance for those who suffer genetic abnormalities should not deter us from taking responsibility for preventing further occurrences of this suffering. (Again, when detection of genetic disease occurs during pregnancy and the question of abortion is raised, additional ethical questions arise that are beyond the scope of this chapter.) For those who have been counseled that they may have a child with significant genetic disease, the burden of proof is on the decision to go ahead with pregnancy.

The Genetic Future and the Future of God

In the dialog from Leroy Augenstein's book quoted at the beginning of this chapter, we observed a mother asserting that to prevent the conception or birth of a defective child is to intrude in matters that should be left to God. In our discussion of ethical issues in genetic screening and counseling we have worked with the premise that God has called us to responsible action in these matters and not to mere passivity. However, that approach does not put the matter of human presumption totally to rest. Genetic screening and counseling are two avenues of eugenic control, among others that are available to us through modern science. In the final analysis, screening and counseling need to be considered in this larger context of our potential to control human genesis. It is the prospect of control that invited human beings to consider potentially dehumanizing courses of action.

Daniel Callahan laments the fact that the conventional ethical principles usually applied to test the morality of new developments in the application of genetic knowledge seem always to permit using the new technology without allowing ". . . us in any fashion to pose larger questions about the nature of human happiness, the most appropriate and valuable direction which science as a whole should take, or to inquire about the best ends to which human freedom should be directed."[30] However, while Callahan troubles over the lack of a larger vision that can inform the ethics of our genetic decision, others are confident that they have such a vision. Joseph Fletcher, the ethicist who made "situation ethics" a household word, believes that it is consistent with the rational character of the human makeup to exert as much control as possible in planning our genetic future.[31] Still others cite the possibility of a genetic apocalypse if we continue to pollute the gene pool through unplanned reproduction. Such a prospect would seem to demand stringent controls on reproduction, in which screening and counseling could play a key role.

In contrast to the advocates of stricter controls in planning the genetic future, Marc Lappé has voiced concerns that such reasoning could lead to coercive, societal restrictions on childbearing. Moreover, he debunks on scientific grounds the notion of a genetic apocalypse due to indiscriminate procreation. Apart from the moral problems that discrimination through public policy presents, Lappé concludes that human genetic systems are simply too complex to lend themselves to control. The genetic "burden" is something that should be dealt with by individual families who must make decisions on procreation. To force those who carry harmful traits to do their genetic duty to society by not having children is dangerous to the moral constitution of society, which should dedicate itself to the care of mothers and children, including the congenitally handicapped.[32]

Lurking behind efforts at increased control is not only the desire to reduce suffering but also the desire of some to perpetuate the optimum human type. For the Christian the ideal of our humanity is the image of God revealed in the Christ. The promise of our fulfillment in that image is in the promise of the future kingdom of God at the resurrection of the dead. It is the promise for the perfection of the whole person and the whole world.[33] In view of the comprehensive character of our future in Christ, revealed in the resurrection of the body, we can regard our attempts to reduce suffering and promote health, in genetics and in other fields of endeavor, as anticipations of the fullness of the promise for the new creation in Christ. Our quest for knowledge and its application for the purpose of health is consistent with God's will for his people.[34] We can expect God's help and guidance as we call on him. We labor in hope.

At the same time, we recognize that, while the promise of the kingdom for the fulfillment of our humanity is revealed and established in Christ, it is not yet consummated; it remains both present and future. While we await the perfection of our humanity and the end of all suffering, imperfection and suffering continue; sin continues. Thus, as we do battle with genetic disease with the weapons of medical science, we recognize, or need to, that we are always also at war within ourselves, our sinful inclinations continually threatening our hold on the will of God in our lives. The presumption of human pride can indeed intrude on God's plan, not because we gain knowledge and apply it in forbidden precincts, like genetics, but because our application violates other dimensions of humanity that God would have us safeguard. That is, when freedom and dignity are compromised by a new spirit of dualism in which the flesh is elevated above the spirit in a desire to control its destiny, we have once again distorted our divinely given heritage as human beings.

The ethic of the kingdom is love. By the grace of God in Jesus Christ the love which is spread abroad through the people of God is a sign of the impact of God's kingdom on our present lives. Love is self-sacrificing. It is ready to set aside personal desire and ambition, whether that is to forgo having a child at risk or to exercise constraints in the public use of scientific knowledge. Love knows no barriers to its care. It embraces the weak and the handicapped as well as the strong. Love abhors discrimination, even as it seeks to reduce suffering, because discrimination divides and the promise of the kingdom is wholeness in body, spirit, and community.

Prenatal Diagnosis: Some Moral Considerations

—————Edmund N. Santurri—————

According to a recent assessment, it is now possible, through medical procedures such as amniocentesis, fetoscopy, and ultrasound, to diagnose *in utero* and with considerable accuracy more than 280 abnormalities of pregnancy.[1] These abnormalities include a range of fetal genetic disorders (e.g., Down's syndrome, Tay-Sachs disease, Lesch-Nyhan syndrome, spina bifida) which, if left unattended, will result in births of children suffering from serious physical and/or mental disabilities of varying degree. Given the current state of medical technology, intrauterine therapy for such disorders is possible only in rare instances.

Under certain circumstances—for example, some cases of spina bifida—postnatal therapy can restore the hope for a reasonably normal life. But much depends in such instances on the affliction's degree of severity, a matter which typically cannot be evaluated at the time of prenatal diagnosis. For a number of afflictions, moreover, postnatal therapy cannot remove the primary symptoms of the condition. Thus medically indicated treatment for an infant with Down's syndrome often includes the administration of antibiotics for complications associated with the condition. Yet Down's syndrome children inevitably suffer from some degree of mental retardation, though with special education they often can achieve a substantial measure of independence and in the largest number of instances do lead relatively long and often happy lives. Finally, for certain afflictions such as Tay-Sachs disease or Lesch-Nyhan syndrome the symptoms are harsh, and there exist at present only minimally palliative postnatal therapies. In the most extreme cases, the destinies of children suffering from these afflictions are comparably short lives marked by considerable physical pain and profound mental retardation.

This general state of affairs has given rise to a number of perplexing ethical questions. For one thing, a pregnant woman whose fetus has been diagnosed positively for any of the genetic disorders untreatable *in utero* faces with her family a decision of enormous moral consequence, namely, the decision whether to abort the fetus or bring it to term, in the latter case for the sake of rearing the child or giving it up for adoption. To what extent, if any, can abortion *for genetic defect* be countenanced from the moral point of view? What quality-of-life judgments inform any answer to this question, and how do such judgments bear on our attitudes toward persons actually born with genetic disease? The question of genetic abortion is arguably the most significant of the ethical problems spawned by the new genetic technology. Nonetheless, the advent of modern prenatal diagnostic methods does raise other moral questions that require serious consideration. For example, under current conditions amniocentesis, the most fruitful of the diagnostic techniques, involves certain serious risks for the fetus. Is the taking of such risks morally warranted by the concern to prevent *possible* genetic defect or to prepare a family for the *possible* birth of a child with genetic disease? Under what conditions? There are also a number of ethical questions generated by proposals to make the prenatal detection of genetic disease a matter of *public* policy. What sorts of moral constraints ought to be placed on a screening program? Who, for instance, should have access to such a program and what will be the moral responsibilities of individual physician and client participants? In what follows I examine these and related issues with particular reference to the question of how Christian theological beliefs might direct inquiry in such matters.

Risks of Prenatal Diagnosis

Discussion of the health-risk factors in prenatal diagnosis has focused for the most part on the hazards of amniocentesis, a procedure designed to detect fetal chromosomal abnormalities and other fetal disorders.[2] This technique involves the withdrawal of fluid from the amniotic sac by insertion of a needle through the mother's abdomen into her uterus. At the earliest, the tap should be performed during the 14th week of pregnancy when there is sufficient amniotic fluid for extraction. From the fluid fetal cell cultures can be developed, and these cells allow testing for chromosomal aberrations such as Down's syndrome, as well as inborn errors of metabolism such as Tay-Sachs disease and Lesch-Nyhan syndrome. In addition the fluid itself can be analyzed for excess quantities of the substance alpha-fetoprotein (AFP), a symptom of anencephaly or spina bifida. If all goes well, results are typically available around the 20th week of pregnancy.[3]

As noted by a recent working paper, the health hazards of amniocentesis include risks to the mother, to the fetus, and to the infant during the newborn period.[4]

Generally speaking, maternal complications, when they occur, are minor. Of more than 20,000 amniocenteses surveyed in an international study, one maternal death was reported to have resulted from the procedure. A more probable health risk to the mother is the possibility of infection (amnionitis), which still occurs in fewer than one out of every thousand cases.

All in all, the risks to the fetus are more serious. First, there is the slight possibility (roughly 0.1%) of injury from the needle, but for the most part the signs of such injury have been nothing more than the presence of skin dimples indicating healed punctures, though there have been isolated reports of serious injury such as the loss of an eye. More important, although there is some disagreement about the significance of the findings, evidence exists suggesting that amniocentesis markedly increases the risk of spontaneous abortion. The working paper cited above sets the risk of abortion from amniocentesis at something under 1% and goes on to note that the procedure may be particularly hazardous in this regard for a class of women who typically submit to amniocentesis, namely, those pregnant women with elevated alpha-fetoprotein levels, the presence of which may be indicated preliminarily by maternal serum tests.

Finally, there is some evidence that the procedure poses special risks for the infant during the newborn period. For example, one study indicated a correlation between amniocentesis and respiratory distress syndrome. At the same time, there is no evidence associating the technique with an increase in stillbirths or infant deaths during the first week of birth. Neither is there any evidence suggesting that amniocentesis adversely affects infant development during the first year of life. Researchers have speculated about the possibility of impediment to long-range mental development due to sudden loss of pressure caused by fluid withdrawal. Yet up to now such speculation has been neither confirmed nor falsified. More generally, the question of the procedure's long-term developmental effects, whether harmful or beneficial, remains unresolved.

Given the hazards noted here, any prudent and morally responsible deliberation about whether amniocentesis should be undertaken will involve a careful assessment of the technique's possible benefits in relation to these potential costs. For the purposes of ethical analysis it is essential to note that judgments based on such cost-benefit assessments are inevitably value-laden, i.e., they presuppose value commitments, which can and ought to be submitted to moral scrutiny.

That such judgments are value-laden is a fact sometimes obscured by attempts to *quantify* the decision-making factors. For instance, medical researcher Laurence Karp has argued that given "a total risk figure of 0.5 percent. . ., the performance of diagnostic amniocentesis is certainly reasonable when the risk of diagnosable disease is one percent or higher."[5] Yet despite Karp's conclusion, a judgment that amniocentesis is "reasonable" in such contexts presupposes a resolution to some basic questions regarding the *comparative values* of what might be lost and what might be gained. Indeed, granted certain value priorities (e.g., that it is significantly worse to risk serious harm to a normal fetus than it is to risk bringing a handicapped child into existence), it might be judged *unreasonable* and immoral to undergo the procedure, even under the circumstances Karp describes. Prudent and moral decision making in this area cannot rest simply on factors which admit of quantitative comparison. *Qualitative* considerations invariably intrude.

What the foregoing suggests is that a reasonable judgment about whether amniocentesis should be undertaken in any given case will depend not only on the statistical likelihood of various outcomes but also on a comparative assessment of competing values, such as the avoidance of suffering and the preservation of human life.

On its face this last claim would appear to be uncontroversial. Yet, interestingly enough, it has been suggested that the values at stake in decisions about the procedure *cannot* be compared.[6] Such values are *incommensurable,* presumably, because they cannot be translated into some common, quantifiable denomination that will facilitate comparison. Thus, Paul Ramsey has intimated, one could never justify undertaking amniocentesis by showing that the decision would promote the greatest good overall, because the calculation necessary for determining the greatest good, a calculation that presupposes commensuration of the competing values, is impossible to effect in principle.[7] Of course, if the values at stake in amniocentesis were genuinely incomparable, then it would also seem to be the case that no reasonable deliberation about the procedure's merits could be engaged in at all, a skeptical consequence left unexplored by Ramsey's explicit discussion. Yet, one can grant a measure of truth to these incomparability claims without abandoning the possibility of rational deliberation altogether. True enough, basic human values such as the avoidance of suffering and the preservation of human life cannot be compared quantitatively. At the same time, it is possible to speak of a nonquantitative ordering of such values, and therefore also to speak of reasonable deliberation in such contexts.

The issue before us, then, is whether risk analyses of amniocentesis decisions yield conflicts among values that admit of some ordering from the Christian moral point of view. Needless to say, there can be no question of constructing an algorithm from which one might deduce unambiguous resolutions for every particular case. The best one can hope for here is the articulation of a general normative orientation that is tied to certain Christian background beliefs and that ought to inform Christian practical reason in specific contexts.

The following set of considerations may serve as illustration. It is commonly proposed that pregnant women who have reached the age of 35 should submit to amniocentesis, the reason being that the chances of conceiving a child with

Down's syndrome increase markedly at this age. Yet frequently this judgment is issued without any explicit comparative evaluation of the stated risk over and against the hazards of the procedure itself. Setting aside for the moment the question whether selective abortion of a Down's syndrome fetus is morally acceptable, we must still ask if the risk of giving birth to a Down's syndrome child is a sufficiently grave reason for taking on the hazards of amniocentesis, particularly the danger of spontaneously aborting a normal child. And when the issue is posed in this way, matters are cast in a somewhat different light. As mentioned earlier, recent assessments set the chances of spontaneous abortion resulting from amniocentesis at something less than 1 out of every 100 cases. At the same time, estimates put the risk of a 35-year-old woman conceiving a child with Down's syndrome at around 1 in 400.[8] Given these figures, the conclusion seems inescapable that a thoughtful judgment supporting amniocentesis and selective abortion for a pregnant woman of this age assumes *ceteris paribus* that risking the loss of a probably normal child would be morally preferable to risking the less likely outcome of giving birth to a child with Down's syndrome.

The point to be stressed here is that this assumption would have a considerable burden of proof to bear, given a moral outlook, such as the Christian one, that characterizes human life as a divine gift and that regards the bringing forth, nurturing, and sustaining of such life as a human analogy to the divine love that issues in the creation and preservation of the world. To defend the assumption, of course, one would need to demonstrate that the life of a child with Down's syndrome is so impoverished in quality or so burdensome to family and society that the concern to extinguish even the relatively distant possibility of giving birth to such a child overrides any presumptive obligation, grounded in Christian ethics, to care for the probably normal child.

It is difficult to see how the aforementioned burden of proof could be borne. This judgment is partially a function of realizing that children with Down's syndrome, though significantly limited in potential and exceptionally dependent on familial and social resources, can with proper care lead flourishing lives.[9] Indeed, granted a moral assumption in favor of sustaining human life, it would seem to be unreasonable, all other things being equal, to risk the loss of a normal child in order to prevent the birth of what could very likely be a flourishing human existence, albeit one that falls short of social expectations and calls for special ingenuity and perseverance in the provision of care.

But in the present context a decision against amniocentesis can rest principally on the recognition that all other things are not equal under the circumstances described, and that the possibility of giving birth to a Down's syndrome child is under those circumstances remote in relation to the risks of spontaneous abortion. As the probability of such a birth increases, the concern to prevent the hardship that ordinarily does attend the rearing of an affected child will naturally gain in significance relative to the concern for protecting the normal child.

For instance, the chance that a woman at age 44 will conceive a child with Down's syndrome is 1 in 35, and at age 48, 1 in 12. The risks are even greater, moreover, for parents who previously have had children with chromosomal abnormalities. Under any of these latter conditions, the less than 1% chance of spontaneous abortion may begin to look like a minor matter. Of course, whether a woman ought to submit to the procedure in cases in which the risks of Down's syndrome are relatively significant will depend on the ultimate purpose in so doing. If the goal is selective abortion given positive diagnosis, then we are left with the question whether such an abortion is morally defensible, a question I shall consider later on. If, on the other hand, the purpose of amniocentesis is to prepare psychologically or otherwise for the possible birth of an affected child, the issue becomes one of determining whether the goods that would be served by such preparation are sufficiently weighty to justify hazarding an accidental abortion.

The general point is that despite frequent suggestions to the contrary, the risks posed by amniocentesis, preeminently the risk of spontaneous abortion, make submission to the procedure an action requiring special moral defense, given an assumption favoring the protection of human life. As we have seen, whether the threat of Down's syndrome is sufficient to carry this defense will depend on a variety of factors, including the relative probabilities of different outcomes and the comparative values of possible losses and gains.

I have focused on this especially problematic case mainly because recommendations of the procedure in this context are typically issued with inadequate reflection on such factors. Yet the special emphasis here should not obscure the fact that amniocentesis can be utilized to detect other genetic abnormalities with different levels of severity as well as different degrees of probable occurrence and that the differences will affect one's moral assessment of the procedure. In the most extreme instances, indeed, the gravity of the disorder, combined with a high probability of affliction, will serve to shift the weight of moral concern *decisively* from the question of the procedure's hazards to the question of selective abortion on positive diagnosis.

Consider the case of Lesch-Nyhan syndrome, a condition whose symptoms include mental retardation, an inability to walk or sit up without assistance, uncontrollable writhing body movements, and compulsive self-mutilation involving the biting of lips, fingers, and shoulders. Those afflicted usually die before the age of 20. The disease affects males only; females are carriers. Although the condition cannot be diagnosed in the carrier state, we know that for a woman who has given birth to an afflicted child there is a 50% chance that a male child of a subsequent pregnancy will suffer from the disease and a 50% chance that a female child will be a carrier. Amniocentesis can detect the presence of the disease in the male fetus. Now it is quite plausible to argue that all possible precautions should be taken to avoid pregnancy after the birth of a child suffering from the condition. But, assuming a subsequent conception, whether by accident or design, it is equally plausible to contend that, if the symptoms of Lesch-Nyhan syndrome are grave enough to warrant selective abortion of an affected fetus (and the argument would seem to be as forceful here as anywhere), then the high probability of the disease's presence relative to the risk of spontaneous abortion makes the choice of amniocentesis a reasonable one. In reflecting on this case, then, one is inevitably driven to consider the moral status of abortion for genetic defect. And, given the current state of affairs, there will be a range of relevantly similar cases, where resolution of the moral issues surrounding the hazards of prenatal diagnostic procedures will depend on prior adjudication of the moral debate over selective abortion.

Genetic Abortion

There likely will come a day in the not-too-distant future when advances in genetic technology will have made intrauterine therapy the standard medical response to prenatally diagnosed genetic disease. Unfortunately, while there has been some progress in this area, that day has not yet arrived. And, until it does, we shall be forced to come to grips with the problem of abortion for genetic defect. Of course, to characterize genetic abortion as a *problem* is not to raise questions about its legality; even postamniocentesis abortion, coming as late as it does in the pregnancy's term, still falls within the legal limits established by the Supreme Court. At the same time, I shall be assuming here that genetic abortion does constitute a *moral* problem, particularly from the viewpoint of Christian ethics. Such abortion is morally problematic, given the recognition of a presumptive obligation on parents to protect their fetuses from harm, an obligation that has its source not in some putative fact that the fetus is an actual or a potential *person,* as some contemporary philosophers utilize that term (self-conscious, autonomous being), but rather in the fact that the fetus is an unborn *child* whose being lays moral claim to parental care. For Christian ethics this moral claim is part and parcel of an objectively real parent-child covenant, which mirrors analogically the providential covenant God has forged with the world. Since care for children typically involves protection against their destruction, this parental covenant generates a moral assumption against abortion. To note the assumption, however, is not to suggest its indefeasibility. Indeed, as far as Christian ethics is concerned, it is fruitful to regard the problem posed by genetic abortion as the problem of determining whether there are conditions under which the moral obligation to care allows a parent to set aside, albeit tragically, the assumption against fetal destruction.[10]

The considerations generally advanced in support of genetic abortion are unquestionably compelling ones.[11] In the first place, the bearing and rearing of a handicapped child imposes extraordinary burdens on the child's family. These burdens often include severe financial hardship, enormous time and energy expenditures that deprive other children in the family of parental attention, significant restrictions on geographical mobility, and, perhaps most important, debilitating emotional experiences, such as profound grief over the affected child's condition, frustrated hopes and expectations, guilt feelings, and a diminshed sense of parental self-esteem.[12] With genetic abortion many of these harmful consequences can be avoided. Second, aborting a child with genetic abnormalities benefits society at large by effecting substantial savings of resources that would otherwise be needed for special care and education and by helping (some would argue) to prevent deterioration of the "gene pool," thereby contributing to the goal of an acceptable quality of life for future generations.[13] Finally, genetic abortion, at least in certain circumstances, might be seen to benefit the fetus itself. As we have seen already, some genetic aberrations detectable *in utero* exhibit a variety of symptoms that collectively make for a life of impoverished quality. Under such conditions, one might argue, it is in the interest of the fetus not to be brought to term.

Formidable as these reasons are, it is crucial for the purposes of ethical reflection to distinguish the first two, which are utilitarian in nature, from the last, which is "patient-centered" in character.[14] The distinction is necessary, granted the premise that the fetus is a child who lays moral claim to care; for it is difficult to see how any genetic abortion other than one grounded in patient-centered considerations could be reconciled with a position that acknowledges this moral claim.[15] Part of what it means to care for a child, after all, is to insure, whenever possible, that the value of his or her existence will not be assessed purely in instrumental terms and that the course of the child's history will not be determined exclusively by purposes unrelated to his or her own well-being. Caring for a child, in other words, involves guarding against the child's being treated simply as a means to the ends of others—whether the ends are those of the family or the society at large.

None of this is to deny that satisfaction of a child's interests often must give way to a more general familial or social concern. Indeed, in certain cases of intrafamilial conflict parental care may require the suppression of one interest for the sake of fulfilling another, more important one. Yet such care also recognizes that, except for the most desperate situations, certain *fundamental* interests of the child must not be sacrificed for the sake of the common welfare and therefore should not be subject to the sort of bartering that marks utilitarian calculations of the greatest good for the greatest number. Among these fundamental interests, naturally, is the child's interest in continued existence. Except for the most extraordinary of circumstances, care assumes that a child's life will not be given up merely because the child's death will serve the needs of others.[16] And if the fetus is seen as a child, then the same stricture would seem to apply here. Given the canons of parental care, genetic abortion will be morally justifiable—if it is justifiable at all—not because it enhances familial or social well-being (as important as such concerns are), but only insofar as it can be seen to serve the interests of the fetus itself.

Of course, it is one thing to press this last claim. It is quite another to contend that certain genetic abortions in fact do promote the fetus's best interests and consequently can be construed as acts of parental care. Nonetheless, despite the strong assumption against fetal destruction articulated earlier, I would propose that some genetic abortions can be regarded intelligibly as expressions of such care and thus are morally justifiable, though I would emphasize also that one must discriminate carefully among cases as well as acknowledge a measure of tentativeness about particular judgments.

I have intimated already that a fetus with Lesch-Nyhan syndrome is a strong candidate for selective abortion, and there are a number of relevantly similar instances. Consider the case of Tay-Sachs disease. A child suffering from this condition appears to be normal shortly after birth but within months begins to show signs of lethargy, weakness, and arrested psychomotor development. Eventually the stricken child is overcome by even graver symptoms, e.g., blindness, deafness, proclivity to seizures, paralysis, and profound mental retardation. Death typically occurs between the ages of three and five. Granted these circumstances, it is certainly reasonable to suggest that a decision to abort a Tay-Sachs fetus falls within the boundaries established by a concern for its well-being, because it is also reasonable to argue that death is preferable to continued existence, from the point of view of the afflicted life. Or take the case of *epidermolysis bulloso lethalis,* a condition which practically limits touching an affected child since such contact frequently results in the formation of large blisters that become infected and require hospital treatment. Once again, it is within reason to claim that abortion upon diagnosis of the disease is warranted precisely by the concern to advance the fetus's best interests. Other examples could be cited. The general point is that for certain genetic diseases detectable *in utero* the prospective symptoms are so harsh that it is meaningful to speak of selective abortion not as the abandonment of parental care but, quite the contrary, as the very manifestation of such care.

At the same time, there are other genetic afflictions in relation to which a patient-centered case for selective abortion is not so easily made—if it can be made at all. Among these afflictions, naturally, are those that admit of postnatal correction (e.g., cleft palate, galactosemia); yet included also are certain genetic diseases that are fairly serious in nature and cannot be cured. Take once again the case of Down's syndrome. Earlier I noted that a Down's syndrome life has the capacity to flourish under optimal conditions, which include, among other things, special care and education. True enough, such a life is substantially limited in potential; some degree of mental retardation is almost always a symptom (though the *precise* degree cannot be established *in utero* or even shortly after birth), and there are often physical disabilities with varying levels of severity, e.g., heart disease and respiratory complications. Indeed, one could argue quite plausibly that a competent, normal person would, if given the choice, elect death over a life lived in these circumstances. Yet it would be a doubtful proposition to assert from the perspective of the Down's syndrome life itself that death is preferable to life. After all, as is commonly observed, children stricken with this condition often appear quite happy. They frequently take pride in their accomplishments, thrive under the rigors of competition (witness the Special Olympics), experience pleasure in bringing joy to others, and form lasting relationships. Given these facts, it would be implausible to suggest that for a typical Down's syndrome child life is *not* worth living. But if this is true, then it would also be hard to argue that genetic abortion would be in the best interests of the Down's syndrome fetus and consequently difficult to construe such an abortion as an informed expression of parental care.

It is important, then, to distinguish the perspective of a reasonable person, who might choose not to suffer a certain affliction (even at the expense of choosing death) from the perspective of the afflicted person himself or herself, for whom life, even with serious limitations, may be worthwhile.[17] Of course, even when this distinction is preserved, difficult choices about genetic abortion remain. One reason for the difficulty is the predictive uncertainty that accompanies prenatal assessments. For one thing there is the possibility of outright misdiagnosis, the consequence of human error (roughly 0.5% of all amniocenteses). Moreover, with some diseases there is enormous variation in degree of severity, and the exact degree in any given case cannot be projected by the appropriate prenatal test. A case in point is the test measuring AFP levels in the amniotic fluid. Excess quantities of this substance indicate with considerable reliability the presence of a neural tube defect, which about 50% of the time turns out to be anencephaly (no brain or substantially undeveloped brain), a condition invariably resulting in death before or shortly after birth. The other half of the time the defect takes the form of spina bifida, a condition in which part of the spinal cord protrudes through the unfused vertebrae. In certain instances the spina bifida wound is inoperable, and the infant will die shortly after birth. In other cases, however, the child can survive, sometimes with therapy and sometimes without, but the quality of life varies significantly depending on the size and location of the defect. Under the best circumstances there will be a reasonably normal life. Under the worst, there will be a number of debilitating handicaps, including enlarged head, mental retardation, paralysis from the waist down, curvature of the spine, excretory incontinence, and meningitis. For present purposes the crucial fact is that no particular one of these outcomes can be forecast at the time of prenatal diagnosis, and this indeterminacy naturally complicates decision making regarding genetic abortion.

In addition to such *empirical* uncertainty, there is also an element of *normative* uncertainty surrounding certain genetic abortion decisions. Again the case of spina bifida provides a suitable example. For even if the worst spina bifida conditions could be projected with reasonable assurance, it would still be difficult to say whether the prospect of these conditions would warrant abortion of an affected fetus. The problem is that despite the unquestionable hardships involved, there is evidence that even in these burdensome circumstances life can be happy and meaningful.[18] Indeed, given a moral assumption against fetal destruction, perhaps the reasonable choice under such conditions of uncertainty (normative or empirical) is to forgo the abortion option in the hope that a tolerable existence will be achieved.

Now in response to all of this, some object that raising the question of *which* burdens make a life unworthy of living obscures a more fundamental problem with the position I have outlined thus far. According to the objection, the really central question is whether *any* potential burden of existence could ever render *nonexistence* a *benefit* to the fetus. The problem presumably is conceptual in nature:

> Ordinarily where we choose to act against abnormality and suffering, we do so on the assumption of the beneficiary's continued existence. In fact, we choose to act against these *in order to* enhance that continued existence. In part we encourage and approve of benevolent and beneficial acts for others because the other will enjoy, experience, and approve the outcome of our choice. Unfortunately this is not possible for the malformed fetus. The available options for *this* existing *conceptus* do not include continued "healthy" or "normal" existence. So the "benefit" of nonexistence and the reduction of suffering it brings for the fetus occurs in the absence of the continued existence during which the beneficiary could experience the results of that choice. Can we speak of benefits without a beneficiary?[19]

If this line of reasoning is correct, then to speak of abortion *for the sake of the fetus* is to wrench a number of concepts from their typical settings and to employ those concepts in ways that risk transgressing the very limits of intelligibility.

Of course, there can be no denying that our *ordinary* assessments of benefits and burdens do presuppose the continued existence of the beneficiary. As John Arras has recently noted, however, there remain compelling reasons for regarding death as a benefit in some circumstances.[20] First, situations involving severe genetic abnormalities are extraordinary in nature and serve to break the conceptual bond between "life" and "good," a bond that typically informs our thinking about human welfare. In these situations, the afflicted is irremediably cut off from the possibility of realizing those very goods that lead us to see life as a necessary condition of any benefit. Second, to deny on conceptual grounds that death could ever be beneficial would be to deny, for instance, that a competent patient could reasonably refuse an extremely burdensome medical treatment necessary to sustain life. Yet most would allow that such a refusal would be reasonable in certain contexts and thus most by implication would grant that death could be construed as a benefit in relation to a significantly impoverished life. Of course, in cases of genetic abortion the judgment in favor of death is one issued by a competent guardian for an incompetent beneficiary. Under such conditions, naturally, special care must be taken to insure that genuine interests are being served. But to counsel caution in these cases is to admit nothing that impugns the *rationality* of talk about abortion for the fetus's sake.

A second possible objection to my general account alleges that a disturbing implication follows from any position that allows for quality-of-life justifications of abortion. According to this criticism, if we permit selective abortion on the grounds that some burdens of genetic disease are simply too great to bear, then as a matter of consistency we must also consider burdens unrelated or at best contingently related to genetic disease. For example, while a Down's syndrome child may flourish under optimal conditions, much depends on the quality of social support available for proper nurturing. Though society has done much to provide the appropriate services, in certain situations delivery systems, unfortunately, remain inadequate. Given this state of affairs, a Down's syndrome child may for a variety of reasons find himself or herself living under conditions that are anything but optimal. Should this fact be taken as relevant to assessing whether a Down's child's life is worth living? Or, if intolerable burden is really the critical issue, why not cast the net more widely to include even those genetically normal fetuses whose lives will be made miserable by social circumstances? Is the prospect of a life in South Africa, for instance, ground for aborting a black fetus? Does being Jewish in Nazi Germany count? If not, then what precisely is the difference between these cases and the genetic abortion being advocated?

In addressing this last question, one might be tempted to reply that abortion of a fetus for reasons of race, nationality, religion, or sex (call this *social* abortion) is unjustly discriminatory, whereas abortion of a fetus with genetic defect is not.[21] Yet this reply misses a crucial similarity between the distinguished actions. Granted, in the case of genetic abnormality the justification of abortion resides not in the mere fact that the fetus is abnormal or genetically different but rather in the fact that the difference will spell immeasurable suffering for the afflicted child. However, similar things can be said regarding social abortions. In these cases, too, the reason for abortion, given the terms of the argument, is not simply race, nationality, and so forth, but rather the fact that the cited characteristics will lead to suffering for the child under the conditions depicted. Indeed, the most that could be said about abortion in such contexts is that it represents, more than likely, too quick a concession to social and political injustice.

But here, I think, *is* the differentiating factor. The instances of genetic abortion I have presented as consistent with parental care are instances in which the prospective burdens are enormous, acute, and most important, virtually certain to be borne. In the cases of social abortion the projected burdens are serious enough, but typically there is hope that the worst of them can be avoided or mitigated. Unjust social structures, after all, can be replaced, modified, tinkered with, protested, and even evaded if need be. Unfortunately, the same cannot be said about genetic structures, at least in the relevant cases. Of course, we can construct scenarios in which the hope to escape the harmful effects of unjust social structures is theoretical at best (e.g., a pregnant Jewish woman in a Nazi death camp where newborn infants are systematically drafted for painful, lethal experimentation). Given such circumstances, one would be hard pressed to deny that abortion was consistent with parental care. But under typical conditions matters are not so desperate. And we can apply this insight to the Down's syndrome example introduced earlier. While social conditions for rearing Down's syndrome children are by no means perfect, there is the hope that through the initiatives of parents and others social settings can be arranged to foster happy, meaningful life. Where there is such hope, life ought to be sustained. Indeed, we can go one step further and maintain that the moral obligation to provide care generates a correlative obligation to create the social conditions which make such care possible.

This brings us to a final criticism of my general position on selective abortion. According to this objection, allowing abortion for genetic defect risks leading society down a slippery slope toward a common disrespect for the lives suffering from these afflictions.[22] A scenario is easy to envisage: The widespread practice of genetic abortion causes persons to regard those affected by genetic disease as beings who are ''unfit to be alive.'' A consequence is that handicapped children who do get through the ''safety net'' of prenatal screening come to be viewed as ''mistakes.'' Parents giving birth to such children see their offspring as beings who ought never to have been born. The children themselves—at least those with sufficient capacity to understand—resent the fact that they have been brought into existence; indeed, they regard their very lives as injuries that ought to have been prevented. A further general consequence is the raising of standards for counting human beings as full-fledged members of the moral community, with the attendant result that the handicapped suffer a diminishment of status. Under such conditions, the provision of care for humans with genetic disease deteriorates, because now such service is seen as a matter of comparatively minor importance. Last, relatively moderate judgments and practices lead to more radical assessments and policies. *Abortion of a fetus for genetic reasons* becomes *withholding of life-sustaining medical treatment from afflicted infants, children, and adults,* and *withholding of treatment* becomes *direct killing of such infants, children, and adults.*

Some argue that permitting genetic abortion risks producing the social transformations depicted in the foregoing precisely because the moral principles that justify such abortion simultaneously justify those very transformations.[23] Yet it is essential to draw attention to an equivocation that commonly forms part of this argument, an equivocation on the concept of worth. It is one thing to say, for instance, (A) that a Lesch-Nyhan life is not worth living, in the sense that it is not in the sufferer's interests to have his existence continued. Such a statement, as I have argued, would be part of any proper justification for genetic abortion. It is, however, quite another thing to claim (B) that Lesch-Nyhan disease so detracts from the sufferer's quality of life that he no longer bears moral worth, no longer commands the fullest moral consideration of the community. (B) does not follow logically from (A); justifying abortion for Lesch-Nyhan disease, therefore, does not lead as a matter of consistency to justifying social arrangements that diminish the moral status of those born with the condition. Of course, society is not always rational, and consequently such distinctions may be missed. For this reason it will be necessary to erect safeguards of various sorts to insure that a policy of genetic abortion will not erode standards according full moral status to human beings who are born with genetic disease.

Having made this point, however, I am also compelled to admit that one potentially troubling implication does appear to follow from the justification of genetic abortion I have presented. The question is whether the principles that warrant abortion for genetic reasons also—as a matter of logic—warrant infanticide for those same reasons in cases where the abnormality has gone undetected *in utero*. Needless to say, this question cannot be resolved apart from settling what is arguably the central issue in the abortion debate at large, namely, the issue of the fetus's moral status. Of course, there can be no denying the descriptive difference between killing a fetus and killing an infant; the question is whether the difference is normatively significant. If the fetus's normative status does differ from the infant's, then there is no inconsistency in countenancing abortion while prohibiting infanticide. If, on the other hand, the statuses are equivalent, then, it would appear, logic compels the proponent of genetic abortion to approve of infanticide when the disabilities are relevantly equivalent.

I have proposed in previous discussion that the fetus is to be regarded as a child who lays moral claim to the parental care owed any child. But, if this is so, and if, as I have argued, genetic abortion can be construed as an expression of such care under certain conditions, then we must be open to the possibility that infanticide, likewise, may be regarded as an expression of such care. I reach this conclusion with considerable trepidation and a host of unanswered questions regarding the harmful social consequences that could result from crossing the psychological threshold separating abortion from infanticide. Indeed, given the uncertainties here and given the judgment of the common moral consciousness, which undeniably assesses abortion and infanticide in different terms, perhaps the *reasonable* course, paradoxically enough, is to heed the dictates of that consciousness and embrace the inconsistency of a practice that accepts the killing of fetuses for genetic abnormality but rejects the killing of newborns similarly affected.[24]

Prenatal Screening as Social Policy

Beyond the moral issues related to individual parental choice about prenatal diagnosis and genetic abortion, we are faced with a series of important ethical questions generated by proposals to make prenatal screening a goal of public policy. In this section I shall address some of these questions, though it should be noted at the outset that the issues are enormous and warrant more detailed treatment than I can give here. For the sake of convenience I shall focus on one of the more commonly discussed proposals: advocacy of a mass prenatal screening program designed to detect neural-tube defects in the general population. Needless to say, I proceed with the same moral reservations expressed earlier about aborting fetuses when such defects are indicated prenatally. Yet, given the current legal state of affairs in which these abortions are assumed to be permissible, it becomes important to consider the proposal with an eye to other ethical questions that have structured the general policy debate.

A mass screening program for neural-tube defect would involve routine implementation of a series of maternal tests currently provided by a number of medical centers in this country and others. The first of the series is given between the 15th and 20th weeks of pregnancy and is designed to measure AFP levels in the maternal blood. Excess levels of AFP in the blood at this stage of pregnancy signify any of the following conditions: (1) a twin pregnancy, (2) a pregnancy further advanced than originally thought, or (3) a fetus suffering from neural-tube defect. If this first test is positive, then the step is repeated, and often the result will be negative. If the second test is positive, then ultrasound is employed to determine whether condition (1) or (2) obtains. If ultrasound fails to detect either condition, then amniocentesis is performed to assess the levels of AFP in the amniotic fluid. An abnormally high level is a fairly reliable indicator of tubal defect, though there is still the slight possibility of misdiagnosis. At this juncture either of two confirmatory tests is occasionally employed—an advanced ultrasound technique, which under optimal conditions can detect spina bifida lesions, or a chemical test for a particular enzyme (acetylcholinesterase) whose presence is associated with tubal defect. Given positive results at this point, the odds are very strong that the mother is carrying an affected fetus. On the other hand, for those women who have received negative results at any stage of the process the likelihood is high that the pregnancy is unaffected.

Still, there are no absolute certainties here. In any mass screening program for AFP, we can expect a number of false-positive as well as a number of false-negative results. What this will mean when such a program is tied directly to genetic abortion is that some normal fetuses that would otherwise have been carried to term will be aborted, and some affected fetuses that would otherwise have been aborted will be brought to term. For present purposes a significant fact is that in setting up an AFP screening program a choice must be made between minimizing the number of false positives at the expense of generating a comparably large number of false negatives or minimizing the false negatives at the expense of producing a comparably high frequency of false positives. If the program sets a relatively high cutoff point for normal AFP levels, then false negatives will be comparatively frequent, and false positives, comparatively infrequent. If, on the other hand, the cutoff point is relatively high, then false negatives will be minimized at the cost of generating more false positives.

Which testing bias is to be preferred? Of course, the answer to this question will depend on how one assesses the values of alternative losses and gains. Granted a connection between AFP screening and genetic abortion, preference for a low false-negative rate suggests the judgment that *ceteris paribus* it is worse to bring into existence unexpectedly handicapped children than it is to abort unexpectedly normal children, and preference for a low false-positive rate suggests the view that it is worse to abort the normal children than carry the handicapped children to term, all other things being equal. As Natalie Abrams has noted, it would be difficult if not impossible to determine which outcome is better simply by appealing to psychological or economic considerations.[25] The psychological consequences for a woman who aborts an unexpectedly normal child would appear to be comparable in severity to those for a woman who carries an unexpectedly handicapped child to term. On the other hand, economic assessments of either bias in test design will vary, depending on the type of expense being evaluated. If the costs of caring for handicapped children are at the center of consideration, then a high false-positive rate would seem preferable. If the concern is for the costs of the screening program itself, then a low false-positive rate would appear to be desirable, because a high cutoff point for AFP levels would minimize the number of women sent on for subsequent tests.

In any event, the importance of such psychological and economic assessments will be subject to question, given the moral stance assumed here. From this perspective screening programs should be evaluated primarily by virtue of their strengths and weaknesses as support systems for parents engaged in the covenantal activity of caring for their children. In light of *this* concern, the central question to be asked is what policy would best serve the fundamental interests of those children who will be subject to the screening process. And even if we concede, despite the moral reservations expressed earlier, (1) that abortion on positive diagnosis of neural-tube defect can be rendered consistent with canons of parental care and thus (2) that screening programs for such defects can be regarded generally as mechanisms of assistance for caretaking parents, it is still reasonable to insist that the uncertainties involved in gauging prenatally the quality of spina bifida life remain significant and, as such, should temper our willingness to risk the loss of *normal* children in order to prevent births of children with this defect.

On this view, then, an AFP program whose testing bias leans in the direction of minimizing false positives will be preferred. Needless to say, such a program should be supplemented by counseling services and other mechanisms designed for the support of women who do give birth to unexpectedly handicapped children as a consequence of false-negative diagnoses or, indeed, for those women who abort unexpectedly normal children as a result of false-positive projections. Regarding this last possibility, it is sometimes questioned whether a physician should spare a women the grief of knowing that she has aborted a normal child by withholding information about false positives. Yet I would argue that despite the very real anguish that would be involved, the woman in these circumstances has a right to such information, particularly because the knowledge gained, in view of statistical probabilities, would be relevant to future childbearing decisions.

In addition to the issue of information availability, the operation of an AFP program raises a number of other sensitive policy questions related to the mutual expectations and responsibilities of individual physician and client participants.[26] For instance, how should a physician respond to a woman who wishes to undergo the screening process but who also announces her intentions not to abort her child under any circumstances? In such a case the physician may determine that

the testing would simply be an imprudent use of valuable resources or an unnecessary risk. Of course, there can be no
question of a doctor submitting to every patient demand, no
matter how unreasonable, and a screening program should be
set up to allow, within limits, for an individual doctor's con-
scientious refusal to perform a particular service. Still, given
the moral presuppositions adopted here, a physician's judgment
on this matter ought to be governed by the question whether
the woman's desire to submit to the tests can be construed
intelligibly as an expression of parental care. Perhaps she is
already the mother of a spina bifida child, is consequently at
heightened risk to give birth to another, and has concluded on
the basis of her past experience that knowing the condition of
this fetus would, in the event of a positive diagnosis, enhance
the necessary preparations for adequate care of the disabled
child. Naturally, it is the responsibility of the physician to see
that the woman's decision is properly informed, that she has
considered, for instance, the risks of the procedure itself. Yet,
if the requirements of informed consent have been satisfied,
then a physician's refusal to perform the tests in such a case
would be morally questionable. At any rate, there is sufficient
reason for holding that a woman's willingness to abort an affected child should not be made a *systematic* condition of entry
into a screening program.

Another problem bearing on mutual expectations and obligations is posed by the woman who undergoes part of the AFP
process with provisionally positive results and chooses to abort
without submitting to follow-up tests. Suppose that after con-
sultation in which she is assured of favorable probabilities and
urged to submit to further testing, she persists in her resolution
to abort on the grounds that she is unwilling to risk even the
most remote possibility of giving birth to a handicapped child.
''The difficult moral question is whether the obstetrician who

performed the AFP test should refuse to perform the abortion, either as a means of trying to convince the woman to proceed with further diagnostic tests or as a statement that he or she will not participate in what may be seen as a misuse of the screening program.[27] One thing seems clear. On the assumption that permissible genetic abortion should conform to certain canons of parental care, the abortion in this case would be morally irresponsible. And an individual physician who shared this assumption should without prejudice to his or her status in a screening program be accorded the right not to perform the procedure in this context.

Whether, as has been suggested, that same physician is morally obligated "to refer such women to other physicians who will perform the desired services" is a difficult matter to assess, despite the undeniable legality of the services in question.[28] From one point of view, such assistance may be regarded as complicity in wrongdoing. From another, it may be seen as a gesture whose purpose is to make the best of a bad state of affairs by insuring that the woman seeking the abortion will receive quality care. Naturally this sort of situation will be especially wrenching for any physician who believes that the moral point of participating in a screening program is to serve parents in the process of caring for their children.

Finally, apart from the issues of test design and individual participant responsibility, the administration of an AFP program raises ethical questions relating to participatory freedom and access. As to freedom, while it is argued occasionally that genetic screening programs offering substantial benefits ought to be compulsory for parties at risk either because the common good will be promoted thereby or because potentially handicapped humans have a putative right not to be born, most would agree that respect for the rights of privacy and individual autonomy demands the establishment of informed consent as a necessary condition of participation. Though in agreement with the conclusion of this consensus opinion, I would add in the way of justification that forcing a woman to submit to amniocentesis and genetic abortion as a matter of public policy would represent an intolerable social usurpation of the prerogative of parenthood, and for *this* reason, if for no other, informed consent should be required for admission into an AFP program. Of course, genuine parental freedom in this area cannot be insured simply by guaranteeing informed consent at the level of entry into the system, because subtle forces may constrain choice at other points in the process.[29] For example, in a society that readily provides support for screening and abortion services but that affords comparatively inadequate resources for the care of handicapped children, there will be enormous pressure on parents not to carry their affected fetuses to term. Similarly, when a health-care system provides substantial support for prenatal screening but inadequate service for abortion, a parent may be compelled against better judgment to give birth to an affected child. Generally speaking, the formal freedoms that most agree should be granted to parents on these matters are of minimal worth unless rendered effective by social conditions that foster genuinely autonomous choice.

The question of who should have access to an AFP screening program naturally cannot be adjudicated without settling the larger questions of the nature of distributive justice and its bearing on the allocation of health care generally. It is a commonly held belief, of course, that health-care services should be regarded as any product is regarded in a free-market economy and that therefore all talk of a *right* to such services without a corresponding ability to pay what the provider demands is as dubious as talk about a right to automobiles under the same conditions. On this view, while society, out of charitable or utilitarian concern, may wish to make screening programs available to all who need them, such is not a requirement of justice, and consequently there need be no injustice in a system that falls short of universal access.

This perception of the matter is widely shared and rests, I am convinced, on some powerful myths depicting medical practitioners and researchers as self-sufficient individuals who, through the free exercise of talent and the sweat of the brow, create *ex nihilo* medical products that by right they should be able to distribute as they see fit. Suffice it to say here that this myth, while deeply engrained, is a fiction—that medical products are the end results of a complex process involving countless contributions (including those of janitors, teachers, bankers, carpenters, spouses, neighbors, and others, in addition to medical personnel) and that therefore medical services can fairly be regarded as social products on which society has just claim.

Given this understanding, how one resolves the moral question of access to a screening program will depend on how one characterizes the social purpose the program is designed to serve. If I am correct in saying that the purpose of such a program, if it is at all justifiable, should be to provide support for parental care, then theoretically the only acceptable condition of access to the system will be the requirement that the applicant be a parent at risk, and thus any restriction based on factors such as wealth or geographical location will simply be unjust. What this conclusion will mean in practical terms for an AFP program is more difficult to say. In ideal circumstances all in need should be served; yet in reality matters are never so simple. Indeed, under certain conditions of scarcity perhaps we would have to settle for a program with limited outreach, where all parents at risk submitted to some just (e.g., random) preliminary selection process. At any rate, whether resources are scarce or abundant, a prenatal screening program that denies those in need an equal opportunity for entry will be a deficient system from the point of view of justice.

Of course, any moral demand for equal access to an AFP screening system will be fully satisfactory only on the assumption that the overall goals of the program are morally acceptable. As I intimated earlier, there ought to be reservations about such goals, because there ought to be reservations about the abortions that the program inevitably encourages. The painful result for someone sharing the fundamental values expressed in this essay will be a divided conscience on many of the policy issues related to the institution and administration of an AFP system. For while there is a responsibility to raise questions in the public arena about a system whose goals are morally problematic, there is also an obligation within limits to maximize the justice of such a system already in place.

The irony is that in seeking this justice one will actually be seeking wider opportunity for participation in an activity one regards as morally dubious. Indeed, I suspect that this sort of tension will inform ethical reflection on many (though not all) of the genetic screening proposals likely to be offered in the near future. At the very least, such moral ambivalence will be experienced by those who believe both that fairness requires equal access to the services society affords and that caring for children, prenatally or postnatally, is an activity that signifies in the created order the divine providential economy at the heart of the Christian story.[30]

Care and Treatment of Severely Handicapped Newborns

—————Hans O. Tiefel—————

In April 1982, in Bloomington, Indiana, a newborn baby needed surgery to repair his incomplete esophagus so that he could eat. His parents denied permission for the operation, and the baby died after six days without food or water. Despite Indiana laws against child neglect and discrimination against the handicapped, state courts upheld the parents in their refusal to permit treatment. Though it seems alarming, this case is not unique, for other children with intestinal blockages have at times also been denied surgery and have died slowly of dehydration and starvation.

What appears as shocking parental and medical negligence become understandable, however, when one adds that these children were all afflicted with Down's syndrome, a disease commonly called "mongolism" because in addition to certain physical abnormalities it results in moderate to severe mental

retardation that is still unpredictable at birth. The physical ob-
struction that prevents eating and drinking and requires surgical
correction—always offered to children who are otherwise normal—gives parents the opportunity in these cases "to let nature
take its course" and "to allow the child to die."

Though not invariably fatal, similar nontreatment decisions
are made for newborns with crippling diseases, such as spina
bifida (cleft spine through which the membranes that cover the
spinal cord protrude), hydrocephalus (accumulation of fluid in
an enlarged head resulting in retardation and convulsions), or
infants who are so immature that they are judged to be pre-
viable. Such children are not born dying, such that their speedy
demise is sure no matter what doctors may do, or that only
palliative care could be offered them. Rather, for a variety of
reasons, they are designated as "nonsalvageable." In what
some regard as beneficent euthanasia, these newborns are not
treated aggressively, and their lives may be deliberately short-
ened through oversedation so that they cannot take their feed-
ings, and thus perish.[1] If these children survive such forms of
"benign" neglect, their subsequent handicaps will be much
greater. The task of this chapter is to analyze and partly resolve
the dilemmas confronting us in such cases of severely handicapped newborns.

In March 1983, the Federal Department of Health and Human Services issued an "Infant Doe" regulation, which in-
sisted that continued federal support of hospitals would require
that signs be posted in every delivery room and nursery stating
that it is a federal offense to withhold food or ordinary medical
care from handicapped infants. Whether one agrees with this
measure, regarding it as a very present help in time of trouble,
as a communal good Samaritan act, or whether one sees it as
Big Brother in the nursery, the question of whether to treat
seriously ill newborns whose diseases have no cure will face
us more and more frequently.[2] For advances in neonatal med-

icine will continue to expand the number of marginally viable newborns who once had no chance at all but who now present us with the dilemma of whether or not to treat them.

This chapter, however, will not describe what can already be done or what may soon be done. Though data about statistics of birth defects, survival rates, symptoms, morbidity, and costs are important, the crucial questions here are not factual or medical, but religious, philosophical, and ethical. My tasks lie first in analyzing the foundations, the ultimate beliefs, on which we base our moral choices. Secondly, this chapter intends to present some Christian guidelines for how to think, talk, and choose when we consider what is right or wrong in our caring for severely handicapped newborn children.

We tend to assume that in matters of moral disagreement, particularly in the pressing and troubling issues on which we cannot come to terms as a nation, the way to proceed lies first in getting our facts straight and then in deliberating the ethical pros and cons. That is a mistake, because diverging moral conclusions often emerge from different visions of what it means to be human and of what life is all about. It is as if those of us who consistently disagree about such issues were seeing the world with different glasses. We look at the same events—seriously handicapped newborns—but they differ in meaning, so we actually see different realities. In such diverging perspectives, facts do not speak for themselves. Closer attention to facts about handicapped children, to their diseases and possible therapies, will not affect the perspectives from which we regard such data. We must instead focus on our glasses, on our philosophies of life, on our presuppositions about what is real and important, before we can understand our disagreement. We must see ''where we are coming from.''

In my judgment persons both inside and outside the church come from different starting points and therefore head in diverging directions. I shall locate those origins, analyze their nature, and inquire how and why they differ. For the sake of simplicity and at the risk of unpardonable generalizing—sinning bravely—I wish to distinguish two different visions that underlie our moral disagreements of what to do about seriously handicapped newborns: *individualistic liberalism* on the one hand, and *a more religious interdependent sense of community* on the other. Though there are a number of overlapping areas in these contrasting visions and though they may coincide repeatedly in their outcomes, I do not believe that these two perspectives are finally reconcilable. Only one can consistently express biblical values and loyalties, though both are usually thought to be Christian. Indeed, they appear to be so interwoven that we have difficulty distinguishing them, that we talk of one in terms of the other, and remain reluctant to acknowledge their differences—even when they pull us in opposite directions.

Individualistic Liberalism and Defective Newborns

By "liberalism" I mean more than a political theory, for it constitutes a worldview, a vision of the meaning and purpose of life. Moreover, liberalism should not be identified with the political left, for it appears across the political spectrum. Liberalist notions of property rights, for example, appear on the far right, while liberalist emphases on civil rights motivate the left.

Liberalism as a worldview conceives of human beings as individual or atomic selves—selves being the locus of what is real and important. Liberalism is at least as old as the Enlightenment and forms a genuine and almost unavoidable feature of our Western self-understanding in that we all tend to begin with the self. Though liberalism has undergone many historical changes, it envisions a reality that consists first and foremost of individuals focused on their own good. It is a creed committed to egalitarianism and individual autonomy. Each person enjoys certain inalienable rights, indispensable to his or her personal self-realization and fulfillment. The civil rights movement and the drive for equal rights for women and other minorities can and do express liberalism at its best: each person counts and should enjoy definite rights or claims for the self with which no one may interfere.

Since individual good, often understood as personal fulfillment or happiness, seems unattainable in isolation, however, individuals form associations, societies, governments. Freely contracting with each other, persons give up some of their liberties for the sake of making life bearable and promising for all. Yet even where persons enter into contracts, such obligations tend to be seen as alien and constraining, threatening all too readily to oppress and enslave. Thus the liberalist suspects government, its power or taxation, its limiting of individual choice. The best government will be one that governs least. And the rights to privacy and to noninterference remain written large in this account of the meaning of life, for such rights protect the value and primacy of persons and resist relegating personal autonomy to social ends or governmental control.

"Liberal" also means "generous," and it seems impossible therefore to fault it on moral grounds. And yet liberalism is not generous toward the unborn or the newborn. Liberalist egalitarianism excludes early forms of human lives from equal consideration; in fact, anything is excluded that cannot sensibly be regarded as a person. To qualify as a person one must have attained at least minimal capacities to reason, to speak, and to relate consciously to others. Only persons can be bearers of rights, since rights are demands against others that must be felt, claimed, and asserted. The unborn, the newborn, the retarded, and the senile remain unable to raise claims or assert rights. The more precise definition of "persons" along rational and volitional lines has become the means by which a number of philosphers have denied equal value, status, and rights to those human beings too young or too old to reason and to choose. Such lives lack equal status and do not count as the likes of us. They would seem to be more akin in worth to property and objects than to members of the human community, so that they "belong" to others who must decide their future. It makes sense from such a perspective to prefer a "quality of life" over a "sanctity of life" ethics for newborns, because nonpersons enjoy no sanctity. In liberalism only persons are sacred, and newborns, as well as some others along the biological spectrum of human life, fail to qualify as persons.

It also appears reasonable in this vision to defer life-or-death decisions about handicapped newborns to the private choices of parents. The lawyer for the child's parents in the Indiana "Infant Doe" case claimed that their decision to prevent their son being treated or fed was a "private matter."[3] The liberalist argues that just as in abortion the unborn derives value only by being desired by its progenitors and loses all worth when unwanted, so handicapped newborns lack claims for consideration when this disappointment—the handicapped newborn—is the last thing the parents want. Liberal abortion laws provide the model for liberalist recommendations for nontreatment of seriously ill, unwanted newborns. "It is reasonable, indeed," a liberalist philosopher declares, "to describe infanticide as postnatal abortion."[4] To be sure, laws still protect all newborns as legal persons, but the law tends to lag behind morality and advances in science. The law seems to be catching up with the liberalist vision, however, when it expands the realm of privacy and refuses, as in Indiana, to intervene in *parens patriae*.[5] A proposal that would bring the law up to date, i.e., conform it to the liberalist vision, is the recommendation to delay legal personhood of newborns long enough for parents to decide whether or not the defective newborn should live. Such legal change might make "it possible to view euthanasia in some instances as a late abortion decision in much the same way that abortion has been viewed as a late birth-control decision."[6]

Liberalism and Language about Newborns

In denying person status to handicapped newborns, individualistic liberalism must take care not to refer to such beings in personal terms. In fact, close attention to language is mandatory for all who speak on the issue of seriously ill infants, for our basic terms reflect and express our vision of who counts and who does not. In this, as in so many ethical issues, how we speak is how we choose. It becomes important, therefore, to see how liberalist language reflects its view of values and of reality. The title of this chapter intends an opposition to a liberalist vision when it uses the word *handicapped*. We use that word for racehorses, but by and large the term applies to persons. As such it does not serve a vision that excludes newborns from personhood. Liberalist writers prefer "damaged" or "defective," depersonalizing terms for things that do not work or turn out to be worthless. Manufacturers' recalls come to mind, and we look for comparative "solutions" to such "reproductive failures" as Down's "cases" or Tay-Sachs "tragedies."[7] The word *newborns,* on the other hand, proves less offensive to the liberal, since most biological reproduction results in newborns and since that term lacks such misleading sequels as "babies" or "children." "Neonate" would probably be the first choice of those who would depersonalize handicapped newborns.

The liberalist linguistic effort to resist any personalizing language that precedes and accompanies personalizing and caring action toward seriously ill newborns meets a natural ally in medical terminology. Insofar as medicine is a science, its language has been cauterized of all personal and nonempirical aspects. Thus medical professionals speak of *fetuses, neonates, biological systems,* and *organisms,* terms that often include us but that we do not apply to ourselves and, in fact, resist outside a technological context. Of course there is nothing wrong with speaking like that in a scientific setting, since medical jargon is merely precise and expert shorthand between professionals. Moreover, though professionals have been known to refer to diseases rather than patients, pediatricians and others who work with newborns tend to use personal names for their patients, a custom that seems to imply person status, though veterinarians may also call their patients by name. When medical language is used by philosophers or laypersons, however, when it becomes the definite language for defective newborns, then such terms obliterate unique value and humanity.

Interestingly enough, when medical professionals use such language in the context of neonatal intensive-care settings, such depersonalizing words are not at odds with the value judgment that handicapped newborns deserve the best that medicine can offer. Or so it used to be. Of late, individualistic liberalism seems to be making inroads into the American Academy of Pediatrics, a majority of whose surgeons who responded to a 1977 survey would agree to withhold lifesaving surgery from children with Down's syndrome.[8] Such physicians "allow their role to shift from that of the handicapped child's defender to his or her arbiter of life or death."[9]

A second indication of moral schizophrenia in the medical community and of support for the liberalist cause in nontreatment of seriously handicapped unwanted newborns is the almost universal use of the term *euthanasia* in this debate.

Euthanasia, or "good death," has been recommended for patients who are terminally ill, for whom death is unavoidable and for whom hopeless therapeutic efforts would be cruel and unjust. However, applying euthanasia to handicapped newborns, who usually are not dying until after they have been declared to be candidates for death, implies that the seriously and incurably ill who are not wanted should be regarded as if they were in fact dying. Though not depriving such newborns of their status of patients or persons, this way of speaking writes off too easily those patients who have a future. Their possible future will be difficult, to be sure, but the dying have no future at all—in this life anyway.

I conclude that while the liberalist vision can be supported by medical language and at times is so used, technical-impersonal and humane-caring ways of speaking are not incompatible in the context of neonatal intensive care. Moreover the very existence of such care argues for treatment of all seriously afflicted newborns. While it is true that some physicians would privatize treatment decisions, arguing that only physicians—or parents and physicians—should decide whether or not to treat, the institution of neonatal intensive-care medicine remains nondiscriminatory, assuming that care should be offered to all unless the patient is too ill to be accessible to care. Furthermore, the professional identity of those who offer care, expressed in the oath of the healer, argues for care for the sick, regardless of whether the newborn is or is not wanted.

Linguistic considerations become significant in an additional way. Advocates of individualistic liberalism also use leading or misleading expressions that appeal universally but actually hide a harsh rejection of unwanted handicapped infants. For example: "Every child has a right to a life free of suffering." Who would or could disagree with that? What parent who has agonized impotently over a suffering child has not tasted bitter injustice? Would that lives free of suffering were ours to grant! But of course all of our lives come without guarantee, though we can at times lessen, or minister to, or share the suffering of others. Yet that is not the intent of that liberalist cliche; instead, it recommends infanticide. The phrase that begins by insisting on the right to life allows only a choice of either life without suffering or death. And since the former is unattainable, the latter must be the only possible choice. Since incurably and seriously ill newborns will never enjoy life free of suffering, it would be best to "allow" or "permit" newborns to die before they become children, i.e., persons. The words *allow* or *permit* also give the impression that one fulfills a request or wish of the defective newborn when one takes its life. Moreover such words imply nonaction, merely allowing events or nature to take their course. But inaction does not forestall moral culpability if we are obligated or responsible for the welfare of such dependents.

Such are liberalist ways of seeing and speaking when it comes to defective neonates, particularly when they are unwanted. When such handicapped offspring are accepted by their parents, on the other hand, nonpersonhood poses no obstacle. And the evaluation of such acceptance tends to be measured in terms of the consequences for members of the family, on how this child creates strains or elicits joys, on how it brings happiness and fits or does not fit into the lives of others, on how it makes individuals into better or worse persons.

Liberalism and Christian Community

Liberalism proves to be so attractive and "natural" that it penetrates the church's self-understanding, its vision or perception of reality, and of course its ethics. For many Christians the gospel resonates with liberalism, since God's redeeming grace also liberates. While not rationally intuited or presupposed, the equal worth of the individual rings true to our conviction that each of us is dear to the Lord. As a child of God each person has individual freedom and dignity. To insist that rights should protect all individuals echoes the prophetic condemnation of exploiting the poor and weak. Civil rights are fitting extensions of Christian love into social dimensions, and equal rights for women acknowledge politically that both sexes are created in God's image.

And yet such blending of liberalism and biblical faith deceives, for it obscures fundamental Christian beliefs about God, others, and the self. To be sure, the liberalist creed yields certain affirmations of personal dignity and freedom that Christians and Jews should support. But the source, nature, and meaning of those affirmations differ when they arise in and express biblical faith. Biblical traditions do not lend themselves to an individualistic starting point in which the rational and choosing self forms the point of origin and prevailing focus. Jews and Christians regard the community of faith and their ties to God as chronologically and logically prior to the self, as values that form and identify who we are. Believers know themselves to be created, sustained, and redeemed by their ties to God and to each other. Relationships with God and each other are not added to the self in voluntary associations; they constitute who we are. To lose them would be to lose ourselves, for without them we could not be ourselves and might not be. If we were able to continue at all in isolation from these life-giving bonds, we would at best be crippled.

Covenant, rather than *contract,* is the fitting word for such bonds, for they constitute the self, remain unconditional, and value others more than self. Thus members of biblical communities learn not to look first to themselves or to make the self the center of their world. They will disavow a liberalist autonomy as alien to those who seek to do their Lord's will rather than their own. They are not pointed to their own fulfillment but to fulfilling the needs of others. In the organic whole that is the people of God or the body of Christ, the welfare of others proves more important than individual self-realization and happiness. Here the question is not how this flawed being, this handicapped newborn, fits into our lives, but how we can fit into its life. Here we do not judge the newborn by its effects on us, but judge ourselves by our responses to its needs. Here we dare not deprive dependent newborns of humanizing and nurturing ties, for without such sustenance we ourselves would shrivel and perish.

Again in contrast to liberalism, the Christian confession that others and we are persons of dignity whose worth should be expressed and protected with rights is not self-evident and does not originate with selves or their rational-volitional capacities. Rather it derives from a source outside ourselves, from a Lord who considers us worthwhile, treats us as dear, binds himself to us, and thereby gives us status. Such standing is not based on what we can or cannot do; it disregards age or merit and bestows itself lavishly on all his children—except that God does discriminate by showing a definite bias for people who are outcast, poor, widowed, oppressed, and (of special relevance here) young and sick.

This divine bias is imitable. God's compassion for the least of his children also urges us who confess to belong to God to see and do likewise. That shared seeing and doing must prevent Christians from joining the debate over whether the unborn or the newborn are persons. If they count for God, how can they not count for us? If the dependence, need, and disability of beginning human lives become occasions for special divine concern, how can believers use those qualities as weapons against them? If God takes a stand with and for them, where do we stand when we exclude them as nonpersons or as non-human? God not only invites us to share his vision; he also holds us responsible for how we see. That awareness of being judged by the measure with which we judge shifts the terms of the debate from whether newborns are persons, bearers of rights, or fully human to whether we will be compassionate, caring, or humane. The inquisitor finds himself or herself placed on trial. Our own status now appears dubious, our own humanity questionable. What sort of persons are we who turn away these dependent creatures by refusing to acknowledge them either as God's own or as our own?

A similar inversion of perspectives growing out of the sense of standing before God in the body of Christ dawns on us when we consider rights in relation to newborns. Not only do rights require person capacities to claim liberties against others (capacities that some dependent human beings lack), but the very idea that rights are the central terms of this issue may be mistaken. Rights focus on what individuals may claim, and divert attention from what we owe them. Those who profess loyalty to Israel's God do not begin with *claims* against their Lord or against one another but with what they *owe* to each. The double love commandment proves paradigmatic by delineating our responsibilities and focusing on our obligations to covenant partners. Within the bonds of genuine community it seems more fitting to ask what we *owe* each other than what individuals may *claim* against each other, even when such rights are raised on behalf of others. The language of rights expresses individualism but may mislead an ethics of community.

A sense of standing in God's and in each others' presence also alters liberalist claims to privacy. To stand before God makes it impossible to consider treatment or nontreatment decisions as private. Here, too, we are called to be the witnessing community. Here, as in all our choices, we are responsible to

God and will never be able to confess that this choice is solely between parents or between parents and physician. When we make such decisions we do not say something only to God but to our children, to members of the body of Christ, and to our neighbors.

Yet surely we would go too far to reject all expressions of liberalism. I have already shown how a biblical compassion for outcasts, the poor, the sick can be expressed in the liberal mode of individual and egalitarian rights. Moreover, liberalism may offer the predominant and perhaps primary concepts or tools for seeking justice in our land. To reject the logic of individualism and its penumbra of rights may well leave the critic without adequate means for pursuing political, economic, and legal justice. But criticism need not imply total rejection. I have focused on the tensions and contradictions between liberalism and the Christian faith in order to resist the liberalist perfusion of Christian self-understanding. Transformation ought instead to proceed in the other direction, for a Christian ethics would want not only to understand the nature and limits of liberalism but should appropriate its virtues and expand the range of those who count in the liberalist vision.

Parents and Children

The nontreatment of seriously ill newborns has misleadingly focused on the person status of these afflicted creatures. Closer scrutiny of the assumptions in looking at their plight in the context of biblical faith not only shifts attention to the decision makers but leads to quite different inquiries. Such refocused questions not only probe our moral identities as Christians but demand a reconsideration of what it means to be a parent and a child.

We tend to regard children as extensions of ourselves. That is accurate insofar as they come from us and we identify with them. We take pride in their achievements and wonder where we went wrong when they fail. Such identification with our offspring may reflect loving bonds with these dear ones, who become more precious to us than our own lives. Or such unifying of self and child may signify that we regard our offspring as ours in a proud and possessive rather than in a self-giving sense. "My" child or "our" child can be lovely words expressing parental devotion, or they can be domineering and selfish terms.

If one begets children to be fulfilled, self-realized, truly happy, if one desires offspring to pass on one's name, a seriously handicapped newborn will frustrate all of those aims to some degree. And if those were motivating purposes for conception, the disappointing outcome of conception appears like a breach of promise. The birth of a handicapped child bitterly frustrates the expectations of a perfect baby; indeed, it shocks parents and elicits psychological reactions of denial, grief, and mourning that parallel the death of loved ones.[10] Depending on our notion of why we have children, the handicapped newborn may become the greatest threat to parental hopes, visions, and plans—in turn threatening the prospects for treatment and the continued existence of the child. Consolation may appear in the thought that one can always "try again," for do not parents have a right to a normal, healthy child? Here the individualistic good of parents remains primary. By contrast, if having and raising offspring is more a matter of creating and serving a child's good, then the disappointment and grief will focus on what the child has lost rather than on the misfortunes of the parents. Then the main concern will be what one can and should now do for the child rather than how to retain or accommodate prior hopes to these stark facts.

At best it is difficult to make life-and-death decisions under the fatigue, stress, and feelings of disappointment that accompany the birth of such children. The feelings of parents in such crises are important, should be taken into account, and probably should be dismissed as sources of moral decisions. Feelings inform us only about the self. They may distort what in fact is happening and what may or may not happen in the future, and they should never be the sole guides to what should be done. The appeal to follow feelings in such crises invokes ethical relativism, in which right and wrong simply express personal feelings and exclude the consideration of what may be good or bad for such children. Such reliance on feelings coincides with the liberal view that offspring are owned by their progenitors, are not yet persons in their own right, should satisfy rather than frustrate parental hopes, and are judged on whether they will fulfill the intent of those who brought them into the world. Here parental expectations and interests tend to conflict with the good of the child, and one may not reasonably expect parents to be reliable representatives or proxies for what such a child would want or for what is best for this offspring.

It may happen that parental rejection of the seriously handicapped child coincides with what is best for that child, for in some tragic cases nontreatment and allowing to die may be the lesser evil for the infant, as I shall argue later. Yet individualistic liberalism insists that only the wishes of parents, informed and facilitated by medical professionals, need be considered. Here privacy forms a fence around parental decisions, a wall resisting all legal, communal, or religious claims to influence or direct their choice. In this view of "defective" offspring, parents claim that this "tragic life" belongs to them alone, for they must live with the consequences of any decision. No one may violate parental conscience or privacy by taking this choice away from them and imposing alien values on those who alone stand to be directly affected by whatever the outcome should be. In this individualistic, the-child-belongs-to-us stance, parents angrily denounce "domineering invasions" and "impositions on their personal plight."

And yet the law tends to deny such parental autonomy and discretion. The legal rights of parents may proceed only in the direction of furthering the welfare and interests of the child. The law offers a one-way street, a ratchet that turns only in the direction of serving rather than of harming the child. When parents misuse or abuse their authority over the child by seriously threatening the child's welfare, health, or even life, the state may intervene temporarily or permanently by depriving parents of custody and by assuming parental obligations to do what is best for the threatened child. An atomistic individualism may well regard such government intervention as morally outrageous and totally unjustified. A more community-conscious and child-centered perspective, however, would endorse the legal assumption that we are our neighbor's keeper and that newborns, handicapped or well, are not extensions or property of parents but constitute our neighbors. Especially Christians and Jews will affirm that we all belong to each other, as well as to God, and that our freedom is not liberation *from unwanted burdens* but freedom *for serving others,* particularly those in greatest need.

Even where parents seek the good of their child first and foremost, their expectations of themselves as parents and their view of the human good may distort the issue of whether or not to treat. We are prone to assume that parents owe their children a fair chance at a happy life. But how can seriously handicapped children ever be truly happy or fulfilled? Or, in the more troubling terms of the liberalist phrase cited earlier, how can parents offer such children a life free of suffering?

Knowing that they will never be able to make such an offer, parents feel hopeless and threatened by the prospect of their child's suffering and may be misled by their own compassion.

> We should never overlook the threat we feel at having to be near those who suffer, even if it is the suffering or assumed future suffering of a new-born. In such circumstances our very humanity can be transformed into inhumanity as we recoil in hate against the other for revealing helplessness. Our very humanity can force us to dehumanize the sufferer.[11]

Caring parents will also wish to offer their children a meaningful life. But if the handicap is serious and debilitating, how can a human life be meaningful? It is true that we admire persons who have overcome their handicap, the individuals with spunk and true grit who heroically surmount incapacitating dependence. Such achievements, like that of Helen Keller, rate high in the American ideals of independence and of the self-made person. (They should rate low among those who confess themselves to be dependent on the grace of others.) It is unreasonable to expect such feats from seriously ill newborns, even when they grow up. Yet meaningful life in our society would call for at least a minimum of independence and social usefulness, of becoming, as we say, a contributing member of society. Whoever does not measure up—and that holds especially for the retarded—does not seem to fit into our society, evoking reactions akin to the ancient charge of being unclean. Even those who dedicate their lives to caring for sick and very dependent children would draw the line at too great a dependence and warn us against making "the unfit survive."[12]

In the perspective of individualistic liberalism, continuing dependence threatens to obliterate any chance for a meaningful life. That may explain the refusal of the parents of Phillip Becker, not a newborn but an 11-year-old boy afflicted with

Down's syndrome and a life-threatening hole in his heart that would kill him painfully by the age of 30 if not corrected, to permit corrective surgery. During most of the five years of legal conflict, courts agreed with the parents, who explained that they did not want their son to outlive them. Though the child had never lived at home with his parents and had been institutionalized since birth—and doing comparatively well—they feared that Phillip would not be well cared for after their death. They not only worried about his quality of life but did not want him to be a burden to his brothers, concluding that it would be best for everyone, including Phillip and the survivors, if he did not outlive them.[13]

Here the issue of whether or not to treat handicapped newborns raises the greatest challenge to Christian self-understanding. How should biblical faith inform our self-conception as parents and our view of what is a reasonably meaningful life for our afflicted children? What is such a life for anyone, especially those confronted with these cruel dilemmas? At the risk of a simplistic confessional response, the fact that God cares for us is sufficient to give life meaning. And that care seems to offer itself in direct proportion to the degree of our dependence. To be sure, God's commandment to love and serve the neighbor may remain hushed or even silent when addressed to the afflicted. But it speaks all the more loudly to the rest of us, who are called to bear each other's burdens, particularly the weight of those who cannot shoulder anything. To expect the disabled to "bear their fair share" or to insist that that is the condition of a meaningful life would signify our unwillingness to recognize the One who sustains us all or to heed his invitation to share that divine load.

In the perspective of faith, the lives of the sick and handicapped become meaningful by being loved by God, a love that also channels itself through parents and other caregivers. The lives of those who are healthy become meaningful—again—by being loved by God and by being asked to become conduits for God's love of his creatures, particularly for those who—in any other perspective—become despised and rejected outcasts. That such caring will not remain free of suffering is one implication of the paradigmatic meanings of the cross. Indeed, if the command to disciples to take up their cross and follow their Lord applies in this context, then we may well have taken the decisive step toward answering the question of what to do in this dilemma.

Handicapped Newborns and Appeals to God

The confession that God shares, and invites us to share, the burdens of the handicapped disregards the spontaneous and seemingly ubiquitous question of why God permits such pain and suffering. The guilt that parents at times mistakenly heap on themselves is here placed on God. Especially in the case of loved ones, we tend to ascribe undeserved suffering to God. "Why did God do this to us?" "What did we do to deserve this?" Such questions assume that these afflictions and miseries must all make sense somehow, and their meaning must be connected with God. To be sympathetic to such questions, it would seem, one should attempt to answer them. In my judgment, that would be a mistake, not because the questions are bad or illegitimate, but because we have no good answers. Bad answers abound, for piety makes too ready use of God in easy explanations and offers cheap theology to get us out of tight spots. It is more honest to admit that we do not know and cannot explain. Moreover, Christian sharing of suffering does not require answers to such questions. Nor does God offer answers when sharing our suffering. Being there, keeping company, helping to bear the load appears to be enough.[14]

Appeals to God as explainer should be resisted, even when they seem to promise comfort. When applied to horrendous, undeserved human suffering, "It is God's will" caricatures as an arbitrary tyrant the One who always seeks to redeem and heal those who suffer. Objectionable kinds of solace also lie in dismissing the seriously ill too readily by pointing to the life to come: "We felt there was a better place for him." [15] That may be true, but before we let him go, we should do all we can to make this place as good for the child as possible.

Sharing the Burden

I have made the case that a biblical faith points in the direction of including handicapped newborns within a community of care and that the greater need of such children calls for more rather than less support. But arguing for saving lives also calls for responsibility for continuing treatment of such lives. There would be little point in keeping such children alive, if one were not to teach them to live, and to live as well as possible. Yet even when they are newborns, the needs of these patients may exceed the financial and emotional capacities of individual couples. The burden such children create and continue to impose is simply more than anyone or any family can bear. If anything proves the inadequacies of individualistic liberalism, it is the dependence of such patients and their families on a wider supportive community. Not only is neonatal intensive care very expensive, but continuing specialized therapy, often lifelong, requires communal help. Health-care professionals condemn the miserly and grudging public support for such programs. They decry the deplorable conditions of state institutions that resemble warehouses or storage spaces more than places of therapeutic care. In the words of a physician who has pioneered in the habilitation and rehabilitation of patients with spina bifida, "If . . . I have preserved a thousand children who are going to sit in wheelchairs in nursing homes with normal intelligence . . ., if that's what I've done, I've created a nightmare."[16]

Those in the pietist tradition will be inclined to offer personal help for the disabled and to support voluntary helping organizations. But a societal commitment to saving newborns requires political and governmental responses to create and finance continuing care. Specifically that calls for a willingness to vote for higher taxes. A conservative reader may find such implications offensive, for liberalism's claim to the almost absolute right to private property has also shaped this facet of the church's thinking. But our resentment over the "theft of tax dollars" may yet be transformed by Christian reflections about stewardship and about our communal obligations to prevent life from becoming "nasty, brutish, and short."

When Not to Treat

This chapter has focused on handicapped newborns, claiming that Christian ethics ordinarily points in the direction of care conceived as treatment. I have neglected the risks of *over*-treatment that result from new technologies, scientific interests, research needs, medical desire to practice skills, parental despair, and institutional inertia. Neonatal care is not immune from the kinds of abuses that have led older patients to insist on living wills and right-to-die laws. Not only mature or aged but beginning human lives may be unreasonably prolonged.

Justification for omitting equal consideration of the risks of overtreatment lies in the fact that—in contrast to nontreatment—overtreatment can be corrected and is not final. Moreover the professional and institutional tendencies to overtreat may largely be a matter of carrying a good thing too far rather than expressing the refusal implied in nontreatment not to extend good things at all. Moreover, the forces making for nontreatment seem more ominous and pervasive than those urging us to do too much. This concluding section aims to redress the imbalance of the earlier too unqualified arguments for treatment.

The fact that this paper has argued for the treatment of handicapped newborns should not imply that such infants should always be treated. A disposition for treatment grows out of the belief that the lives of all children are dear to God and should be dear to us as well. But the immeasurable value of these afflicted lives may be completely and permanently overshadowed by disease, pain, and suffering. The very preciousness of these children may compel us to cease treating when our intervening will no longer do them any good, when our therapies become fruitless and therefore cruel. We must cease when life and continued treatment become so burdensome for these infants that our best efforts will not help to make them better. When treatment ''cannot be conveyed, it need not be extended.''[17] However, we still owe even these children whom we are about to lose our care and our company until they are lost.

Certain diseases may make any treatment senseless from the start. Anencephalic infants (congenital absence of the brain) are never alive, in a sense, because they are already brain dead. Babies with Lesch-Nyhan syndrome (physical and mental retardation, compulsive self-mutilation of fingers and lips, spastic cerebral palsy) are always past cure and soon beyond our help. Even where treatment has begun, as in very low birth weight babies, complications and continuing deterioration will make it necessary and morally right to stop at some point when to continue treating would be to mistreat.

To illustrate the need to stop, this paper concludes as it started, with a case of a newborn with Down's syndrome—the case of Brian West. This newborn also could not be fed because he was born without an esophagus, and his parents, too, refused to consent to surgery. But in this case the state intervened, performed the operation, and two years later, on November 30, 1982, returned custody to the parents. At that time, however, Brian remained hospitalized in intensive care, weighed only 15 pounds, and was fed intravenously and by a tube stuck into his abdomen, because the esophagus reconstructed out of tissue from his stomach was too scarred and swollen to permit swallowing food. Brian died on December 22, 1982, having lost another pound, having never learned to walk, talk, or eat. In addition to two major operations, he had one heart failure, collapsed veins, repeated failures to breathe, and he endured regular antibiotic injections.[18]

It was clearly time to stop, and Brian died without the sort of heroic lifesaving measures that kept him alive earlier. The father was surely right in deeming this death best for Brian. But so was the initial treatment—until this boy no longer could be helped. Our reasons for stopping treatment of handicapped newborns must hold across the life span. No one should be treated when it no longer does any good. That reason does not single out unwanted infants as nonpersons, it does not regard early human life as dispensable or replaceable, and it does not prefer the rights or values of families to the lives and needs of patients.

Notes

Chapter 1   Artificial Insemination

1. Donald P. Goldstein, "Artificial Insemination by Donor— Status and Problems," in *Genetics and the Law,* ed. Aubrey Milunsky and George J. Annas (New York and London: Plenum Press, 1975). See also Richard P. Richards, "Ethical and Theological Aspects," *Soundings* 54, no. 3 (Fall 1971): 315.

2. Martin Curie-Cohen, Leslie Luttrell, and Sander Shapiro, "Current Practice of Artificial Insemination by Donor in the United States," *New England Journal of Medicine* 300, no. 11 (March 1979): 588, and Lucinda Ann Smith, "Artificial Insemination: Disclosure Issues," *Columbia Human Rights Law Review* 11, no. 63 (Spring/Summer 1979): 89-90. See also S. J. Berman and Robert W. Kistner, eds., *Progress in Infertility* (Boston: Little, Brown and Company, 1968), p. 718.

3. Laurelle H. Kinney, "Legal Issues of the New Reproductive Technologies," *California State Bar Journal* 52, no. 6 (Nov.-Dec., 1977): 514.

4. Quoted in Jeffrey M. Shaman, "Legal Aspects of Artificial Insemination," *Journal of Family Law* 18, no. 2 (1979-1980): 333.

5. Ibid., p. 334.

6. Ibid., p. 336.

7. Kinney, p. 515.

8. See Shaman, pp. 336-37; Kinney, p. 515; and John B. Gordon, "Some Legal Considerations," *Soundings* 54, no. 3 (Fall 1971): 312.

9. Shaman, pp. 347-48.

10. Cited by Donald A. Goss, "Current Status of Artificial Insemination with Donor Semen," *American Journal of Obstetrics and Gynecology* 122, no. 2 (May 15, 1975): 248. See also Berman and Kistner, p. 715.

11. Shaman, p. 348.

12. Gordon, p. 313.

13. Berman and Kistner, p. 719.
14. Karl Ostrom, "Psychological Considerations in Evaluating A.I.D.," *Soundings* 54, no. 3 (Fall 1971): 293.
15. Bernard Häring, *Ethics of Manipulation* (New York: Seabury Press, 1975), p. 197.
16. Editor's Introduction, "Artificial Insemination: A Simple Medical Technique, A Complex Human Problem," *Soundings* 54, no. 3 (Fall 1971): 288. See also Robert T. Francoeur, *Utopian Motherhood: New Trends in Human Reproduction* (South Brunswick and New York: A. S. Barnes and Co., 1970), p. 37.
17. Ostrom, p. 296.
18. Ibid.
19. Shaman, p. 331.
20. Lucinda Ann Smith, pp. 92-93.
21. Curie-Cohen, et al., p. 589.
22. Ibid., p. 587.
23. Ibid., p. 585.
24. Ibid., p. 588.
25. George J. Annas, "Artificial Insemination: Beyond the Best Interests of the Donor," *Hastings Center Report* 9, (August 1979): 14.
26. "The Nobel Sperm Bank: An Affront to Humanism," *Humanist* 40, no. 4 (July-Aug. 1980): 61.
27. Joseph Fletcher, *Morals and Medicine* (Princeton, N.J.: Princeton University Press, 1954), p. 139.
28. Ibid., p. 117.
29. Paul Ramsey, *Fabricated Man: The Ethics of Genetic Control* (New Haven and London: Yale University Press, 1970), p. 32.
30. Ibid., p. 33.
31. Ibid., p. 34.
32. Ibid., p. 41.
33. Ibid., p. 44.
34. Ibid., pp. 38-39.
35. Helmut Thielicke, *The Ethics of Sex,* trans. John W. Doberstein (New York: Harper & Row, 1964), p. 259.
36. Ibid., p. 262.

37. Harmon L. Smith, *Ethics and the New Medicine* (Nashville and New York: Abingdon Press, 1970), p. 81.

38. Ibid., p. 84.

39. Pope Pius XII, "To Catholic Doctors," *The Catholic Mind* 48, no. 1048 (April 1950): 252.

40. Karl Rahner, "The Problem of Genetic Manipulation," in *Theological Investigations, Vol. 9: Writings of 1965-67 (1),* trans. Graham Harrison (New York: Herder & Herder, 1972), p. 246.

41. Ramsey, p. 133.

42. Harmon L. Smith, p. 84.

Chapter 2   On Having Children: A Theological and Moral Analysis of *In Vitro* Fertilization

1. Stanley Hauerwas, in testimony before the Ethics Advisory Board of the Department of Health, Education, and Welfare, notes the bizarre character of a society that approves of aborting unwanted children at the same time as it develops an extraordinary procedure such as IVF to provide some women with the experience of pregnancy. The issue, which our society has not been able to articulate with any consistency, is the meaning of childbearing. Hauerwas' testimony and that of others cited in these pages can be secured from the National Technical Information Service in Washington, D.C.

2. Quoted in "Report and Conclusions: HEW Support of Research Involving Human *In Vitro* Fertilization and Embryo Transfer," Ethics Advisory Board, HEW (May 4, 1979): 37.

3. Hauerwas' argument proceeds within a slightly different context from the one I am sketching in these pages, but his question appears to me to be on target. His frame of reference is the Christian community, leading him to develop his answer to the question in a slightly different manner as he relates it to the purpose and goals of Christian community. His discussion appears in the testimony cited in n. 1.

4. Leon R. Kass, "Making Babies—The New Biology and the 'Old Morality,' " *Public Interest* 26 (Winter 1972): 29-30.

5. This kind of critique has been eloquently made by Paul Ramsey. See his ''Shall We 'Reproduce'?'' *Journal of the American Medical Association* 220, nos. 10-11 (June 5 and 12, 1972): 1346-50, 1480-85.

6. Joseph Fletcher, *The Ethics of Genetic Control: Ending Reproduction Roulette* (Garden City, N.Y.: Doubleday, 1974), p. 36.

7. The prerequisites set for IVF patients by the clinic in Norfolk, Virginia, restrict them not only to childless, infertile couples but to married couples whose marriage gives evidence of stability. The stipulated reasons for infertility insure at least the possibility of the couple having their own child, and the woman's uterus must be normal so that she will be capable of bearing her own child.

8. Curran made this point in his testimony before the Ethics Advisory Board of HEW.

9. Warren T. Reich, ed., *Encyclopedia of Bioethics*, vol. 4 (New York: Free Press, 1978), p. 1450.

10. There has been one instance (in Australia) of a normal pregnancy and birth involving an embryo that had been frozen—in this case, for four months.

11. *Christian Century* 99 (January 1982): 79.

12. Arguments in favor of and opposed to federal funding as heard by the Ethics Advisory Board are cited in its ''Report and Conclusions,'' pp. 82ff.

13. Part of the problem now is that certain practices have already been initiated—for example, in the use of sperm banks—that many in our society may want to prohibit. The developments in medical technology go on, but the discussion of their moral implications fails to keep pace.

Chapter 3   Surrogate Motherhood

1. For a firsthand description of surrogate motherhood as it has come to be practiced in the United States, see Noel P. Keane with Dennis L. Breo, *The Surrogate Mother* (New York: Everest House, 1981). Keane is the lawyer who came to prominence for arranging surrogate agreements.

2. These may include inovulation, severe endometriosis, scarred or absent fallopian tubes, or a general medical condition, such as diabetes, that makes pregnancy dangerous or impossible.

3. See the story of Debbie, George, and their surrogate, Sue, who was Debbie's friend, in Keane, Chap. 3. Sue moved in with the couple after the birth of the baby, but did not remain.

4. The artificial insemination need not be performed by a physician. When cooperative physicians could not be located by Keane's clients, the surrogate or the wife of the potential father inseminated the surrogate (Keane, passim). This reemphasizes the point that surrogate motherhood is not a complicated medical process.

5. Walter Wadlington, "Artificial Conception: The Challenge to Family Law," *Virginia Law Review* 69, 3 (April 1983): 479-482.

6. Keane, pp. 234-240, 273, 289, 305.

7. Keane seems to be very careful to inform surrogates of potential hazards. See the "Agreement of Understanding," the "Surrogate Mother Application," and the "Release and Hold Harmless Agreement," reprinted in *The Surrogate Mother*, pp. 275-305.

8. William Graham Cole, *Sex and Love in the Bible* (New York: Association Press, 1959), p. 275.

9. Karen Lebacqz, ed., *Genetics, Ethics and Parenthood* (New York: Pilgrim Press, 1983), pp. 16-23.

10. They may choose never to procreate as a way of avoiding genetically transmitted illness, but they may not use amniocentesis and abortion as ways of "controlling" genetic ills.

11. See Sidney Callahan's provocative article, "An Ethical Analysis of Responsible Parenthood," *Birth Defects: Original Article Series* 15, no. 2 (1979) pp. 224-229.

12. Richard A. McCormick, "Genetic Medicine: Notes on the Moral Literature," *Theological Studies* 33, no. 3 (September 1972): 551.

13. Joseph Fletcher, *The Ethics of Genetic Control* (Garden City, N.Y.: Doubleday, 1974), p. 144.

14. The lack of sexual intercourse is also significant.

15. Stanley Hauerwas is well known for this position regarding other reproductive technologies such as *in vitro* fertilization. See his testimony, "Theological Reflections on IVF" in the Ethics Advisory Board document, *Appendix: HEW Support of Research Involving Human In Vitro Fertilization and Embryo Transfer,* May 4, 1979.

16. Joseph Fletcher and others who might fall under the "spiritualist" label would deny that physical loving communion is necessarily linked to procreation, emphasizing instead the joint *decision* to procreate— by means that may involve others in the physical transmission of life.

17. If the relationship were substantially similar to a marital one, the surrogate arrangement would likely collapse, as would the marriage.

18. The need to develop regulations regarding various kinds of artificial conception, regulations that might be similar to those currently applicable in adoption, is acknowledged in Wadlington, pp. 501-512.

19. Some vocations entail a willingness to sacrifice oneself for another, but these are special cases created by special duties.

Chapter 4   Genetic Manipulation

1. Cf. James M. Gustafson, *Christ and the Moral Life* (New York: Harper and Row, 1968), p. 240.

2. Liebe Cavalieri, "We Do Not Have the Wisdom," *Imprimis,* June 1983, p. 6.

3. Richard N. Ostling, "Scientists Must Not Play God," *Time,* 20 June 1983, p. 67.

4. Jeremy Rifkin, *Algeny* (New York: Viking Press, 1983).

5. Peter Dorfman, "The Rifkin Resolution: Less Than Meets the Eye," *Genetic Engineering News,* July/August 1983.

6. Ibid.

7. Ibid.

8. Ostling, p. 67.

9. "Skeptical Eye," *Discover,* August 1983, p. 6.

10. Alexander Capron, "Enormous Potential for Good," *Imprimis,* June 1983, p. 4.

11. Jonathan D. Moreno, "Private Genes and Public Ethics," *Hastings Center Report* 13 (October 1983): 6.

12. Much of this historical survey is heavily dependent on my previously published article, "Creation in Our Own Image: Ethical Questions," *Christian Century,* 13 September 1978, pp. 818-822.

13. John S. DeMott, "Test-Tube Life: Reg. U.S. Pat. Off.," *Time,* 30 June 1980, p. 52.

14. Alexander Capron, "Looking Back at the President's Commission," *Hastings Center Report* 13 (October 1983): 9.

15. Albert Gore (D., Tenn.), chair of the House Subcommittee on Investigations and Oversight of the Committee on Science and Technology, introduced on April 27, 1983, a bill to establish a new President's Commission that would address genetic engineering in humans. Cf. Moreno, *Hastings Center Report* 13 (October 1983): 5.

16. "New Life Forms: A Clear Road Ahead?" *U.S. News and World Report,* 30 June 1980, p. 35.

17. Paul Preuss, "The Shape of Things to Come," *Science,* December 1983, p. 81.

18. Ibid.

19. Ibid.

20. For a concise statement of the current situation in the genetic engineering of plant life (or "agrigenetics"), cf. *Discover,* December 1983, pp. 88-92.

21. Paul Schimmel, "Genetic Engineering: Blessing or Curse?" *Christianity Today,* 2 June 1978, pp. 15ff.

22. Fay Angus, "The Promise and Perils of Genetic Meddling," *Christianity Today,* 8 May 1981, pp. 26-29.

23. Jonathan King, "Prospects and Hazards of New Genetic Technologies," *Christianity and Crisis,* 19 October 1979, pp. 247-252.

24. Cf. Daniel Callahan, "The Moral Career of Genetic Engineering," *Hastings Center Report,* April 1979, pp. 9, 21.

25. This section is taken from my previously published article, "Creation in Our Own Image: Christian Perspectives," *Christian Century,* 20 September 1978, pp. 855-858.

Chapter 5   Genetic Screening and Counseling

1. Leroy Augenstein, *Come, Let Us Play God* (New York: Harper and Row, 1969), p. 16.
2. Ibid., p. ix.
3. See Rom. 8:18-23.
4. *Newsweek,* 18 May 1981, p. 120.
5. George J. Annas and Brian Coyne, " 'Fitness' for Birth and Reproduction: Legal Implications of Genetic Screening," *Family Law Quarterly* 9 (Fall 1975): 466.
6. *Newsweek,* 18 May 1981, p. 124.
7. Ibid.
8. "Genetic Counseling," March of Dimes Birth Defects Foundation (White Plains, N.Y., 1980), pp. 15-16.
9. Ibid., p. 16.
10. Annas and Coyne, p. 469.
11. Barton Childs, "Prospects for Genetic Screening," *Journal of Pediatrics* 87 (December 1975):1130-31.
12. Annas and Coyne, p. 485.
13. Ibid.
14. Madeleine J. Goodman and Lenn E. Goodman, "The Overselling of Genetic Anxiety," *Hastings Center Report* 13 (October 1982): 20.
15. Ibid., p. 24.
16. Ibid., p. 25.
17. Marc Lappé, James M. Gustafson, et al. "Ethical Issues in Screening for Genetic Disease," *New England Journal of Medicine* 286 (May 1972): 1131.
18. Ibid.
19. Y. Edward Hsia, "The Law and Operation of Genetic Screening Programs," *Genetics and the Law,* vol. 2, ed. Aubrey Milunsky and George J. Annas (New York: Plenum, 1980), p. 111.

20. Paul Ramsey, "Screening: An Ethicists's View," in *Ethical Issues in Human Genetics*, ed. Bruce Hilton et al. (New York and London: Plenum Press, 1973), p. 151.

21. See John A. Osmundsen, "We Are All Mutants—Preventive Genetic Medicine: A Growing Clinical Field Troubled by a Confusion of Ethicists," and Marc Lappé's response, "Mass Genetic Screening Programs and Human Values: Another View," *Medical Dimensions*, February 1973, pp. 5-8, 26-28.

22. I am indebted to Dr. Annamarie Sommer, a geneticist at Children's Hospital, Columbus, Ohio, for this information and for her generous personal interview regarding a number of questions touched on in this study.

23. Aubrey Milunsky and Philip Reilly, "The 'New' Genetics: Emerging Medicolegal Issues in the Prenatal Diagnosis of Hereditary Disorders," *American Journal of Law and Medicine* 1 (March 1975): 73-74. F. Clarke Fraser, "Survey of Counseling Practices," *Ethical Issues in Human Genetics*, pp. 11-12.

24. See the discussion of autonomy and paternalism in James F. Childress, *Priorities in Biomedical Ethics* (Philadelphia: Westminster, 1981), pp. 17-33.

25. For a helpful discussion of this question, see Jay Katz, "Disclosure and Consent," *Genetics and the Law*, vol. 2, pp. 121-129; also: Margery W. Shaw, "Genetic Counseling," *Science* 184, 17 May 1974, p. 751, and David Brock's discussion in *Ethical Issues in Human Genetics*, pp. 91-92.

26. See M. Wayne Clark, "The Pastor as Genetic Counselor," *Journal of Religion and Health* 20 (Winter 1981): 317-332.

27. "The Threat of Hemophilia," Case Studies in Bioethics, *Hastings Center Report* 4 (April 1974): 8.

28. Ibid., pp. 9-10.

29. Charles Birch and Paul Abrecht, ed., *Genetics and the Quality of Life* (Australia: Pergamon Press, 1975), pp. 15-16, 51.

30. Daniel Callahan, "The Moral Career of Genetic Engineering," *Hastings Center Report* 9 (April 1979): 9, 21.

31. Joseph Fletcher, "Ethical Aspects of Genetic Controls," *New England Journal of Medicine* 285 (September 1971):776-783.

32. Marc Lappé, "Moral Obligations and the Fallacies of 'Genetic Control,' " *Theological Studies* 33 (September 1972):411-427.
33. I have developed the biblical, eschatological doctrine of the image of God in *Christian Anthropology and Ethics* (Philadelphia: Fortress Press, 1978).
34. See James M. Childs Jr., "A Theology of Health Care," *Lutheran Standard* 21, no. 5 (6 March 1981): 27-28.

Chapter 6   Prenatal Diagnosis: Some Moral Considerations

1. John Fletcher, *Coping with Genetic Disorders: A Guide for Clergy and Parents* (San Francisco: Harper & Row, 1982), pp. 184-89.
2. Recently, however, questions have been raised about the safety of ultrasound. See Barbara Bolson, "Question of Risk Still Hovers over Routine Prenatal Use of Ultrasound," *Journal of the American Medical Association* 247 (April 1982): 2195-97.
3. A relatively new technique involving chorion sampling is now beginning to provide diagnostic results much earlier in the pregnancy's term. Indications are, however, that the risks of the technique are comparable to those of amniocentesis described below. For a general account of the chorion sampling process see A. V. Cadkin, et al., "Chorionic Villi Sampling: A New Technique for Detection of Abnormalities in the First Trimester," *Radiology* 151 (April 1984): 159-62.
4. Duane Alexander, "Workgroup Paper: Risks of Amniocentesis," in *Maternal Serum Alpha-Fetoprotein: Issues in the Prenatal Screening and Diagnosis of Neural Tube Defects,* ed. Barbara Gastel et al. (Washington, D.C.: U.S. Government Printing Office, 1980), pp. 20-24. Most of the information on risks has been taken from this paper. See also the landmark American, Canadian, and British studies: NICHD National Registry for Amniocentesis Study Group, "Midtrimester Amniocentesis for Prenatal Diagnosis: Safety and Accuracy," *Journal of the American Medical Association* 236 (1976): 1471-76; Nancy E. Simpson et al., "Prenatal Diagnosis of Genetic Disease in Canada: Report of a Collaborative Study," *Canadian Medical*

Association Journal 115 (1976): 739-48; MRC Working Party on Amniocentesis, "An Assessment of the Hazards of Amniocentesis," *British Journal of Obstetrics and Gynecology* 85: supplement no. 2 (1978): 1-41.

5. Laurence E. Karp, "The Prenatal Diagnosis of Genetic Disease," in *Biomedical Ethics,* ed. Thomas A. Mappes and Jane S. Zembatty (New York: McGraw-Hill, 1981), p. 460.

6. Paul Ramsey, "Screening: An Ethicist's View," in *Ethical Issues in Human Genetics,* ed. Bruce Hilton et al. (New York and London: Plenum Press, 1973), pp. 147-61, esp., 151-56. For a more systematic defense of the incommensurability of basic values see Thomas Nagel, *Mortal Questions* (London, New York, and Melbourne: Cambridge University Press, 1979), pp. 128-41.

7. Ramsey, pp. 153, 155.

8. U.S. Department of Health and Human Services, *Amniocentesis for Prenatal Chromosomal Disorders* (Atlanta: Public Health Service, Center for Disease Control, 1980), p. 15.

9. See David F. and Victoria S. Allen, *Ethical Issues in Mental Retardation* (Nashville: Abingdon, 1979), p. 51.

10. Needless to say, this view of the fetus's moral status and the general stance on abortion are both controversial, but neither can be defended at length here. For an extended exploration of the notion that the fetus is an unborn child see William Werpehowski, "The Pathos and Promise of Christian Ethics: A Study of the Abortion Debate" (unpublished paper).

11. John Fletcher, "Prenatal Diagnosis: Ethical Issues," in *Encyclopedia of Bioethics* vol. 3 (New York: Macmillan, 1978), pp. 1330-41.

12. For an insightful account of these effects see John Fletcher, "Attitudes Toward Defective Newborns," *Hastings Center Studies* 2 (January 1974): 21-32.

13. For a version of the gene-pool argument see James V. Neel "Ethical Issues Resulting from Prenatal Diagnosis," in *Early*

Diagnosis of Human Genetic Defects: Scientific and Ethical Considerations, ed. Maureen Harris (Bethesda, Md.: National Institutes of Health, 1971), pp. 219-29.

14. I borrow this phrase from Paul Ramsey. See *The Patient as Person: Explorations in Medical Ethics* (New Haven and London: Yale University Press, 1970), p. 116. Though there are important differences, my general account of care is indebted to Ramsey's account of "covenant fidelity" as expressed throughout this book and in *Ethics at the Edges of Life: Medical and Legal Intersections* (New Haven and London: Yale University Press, 1978).

15. This judgment does not include genetic abortion under *extreme* conditions of choice, e.g., when carrying the fetus to term would endanger the mother's life.

16. By *extraordinary* circumstances I have in mind situations such as the one depicted in the film *Sophie's Choice.* In the title scene the heroine is asked by a sadistic Nazi to choose which of her children is to be separated from her and sent to the death camps. If she refuses to choose, she will lose *both* of them.

17. I owe this distinction to John D. Arras. See "Toward an Ethic of Ambiguity," *Hastings Center Report* 14 (April 1984): 25-33.

18. As the remarks of Dr. R. B. Zachary suggest: "There is no doubt that those who are severely affected at birth will continue to be severely handicapped. But I conceive it to be my duty to overcome that handicap as much as possible and to achieve the maximum development of their potential in as many aspects of life as possible—physical, emotional, recreational, and vocational—and I find them very nice people. . . . Some have been regarded as living completely miserable and unhappy lives. Yet when I see them I find them happy people who can respond to their personal welfare." R. B. Zachary, "Life with Spina Bifida," in *Contemporary Issues in Bioethics,* ed. Tom L. Beauchamp and LeRoy Walters, 2nd ed. (Belmont, Calif.: Wadsworth, 1982), p. 358.

19. Paul F. Camenisch, "Abortion: For the Fetus's Own Sake?" *Hastings Center Report* 6 (April 1976): 39.

20. Arras, "Toward an Ethic of Ambiguity," p. 26.
21. John Arras appears to embrace such a position, though his concern is not abortion but the withholding of neonatal intensive care (ibid., p. 28).
22. See Ramsey, "Screening: An Ethicists's View," pp. 158-160, as well as Leon Kass, "Implications of Prenatal Diagnosis for the Human Right to Life," in *Ethical Issues in Human Genetics,* ed. Hilton et al., pp. 185-89.
23. Kass, p. 191.
24. Whether such a practice should allow for withholding life-sustaining treatment while prohibiting direct killing is a matter I leave open.
25. Natalie Abrams, "Workgroup Paper: Ethical Issues in MSAFP Screening Programs," in *Maternal Serum Alpha-Fetoprotein,* ed. Gastel et al., pp. 74-75.
26. Ibid., pp. 73-74.
27. Ibid., p. 73.
28. Ibid., p. 74.
29. Leroy Walters, "Ethical Perspectives on Maternal Serum Alpha-Fetoprotein Screening," in *Maternal Serum: Alpha-Fetoprotein,* ed. Gastel et al., pp. 69-70.
30. I am indebted to Edward Langerak and Rachel D. Santurri for helpful conversations bearing on the contents of this essay.

Chapter 7   Care and Treatment of Severely Handicapped Newborns

1. C. Everett Koop, "Ethical and Surgical Considerations in the Care of the Newborn with Congenital Abnormalities," in Dennis J. Horan and Melinda Delahoyde, eds., *Infanticide and the Handicapped Newborn* (Provo, Utah: Brigham Young University Press, 1982), p. 99.
2. Gordon B. Avery, "Big Brother in the Nursery," *Washington Post*, 23 March 1983, A 25.
3. Richard A. McCormick, s.j., and Laurence H. Tribe, "Infant Doe: Where to Draw the Line," *Washington Post*, 27 July 1982, A 15.

4. Joseph Fletcher, *Humanhood* (Buffalo, N.Y.: Prometheus Books, 1979), p. 144.

5. "Familial privacy has received increasing protection from law throughout this century" (President's Commission for the Study of Ethical Problems in Medicine and Biomedical and Behavioral Research, *Deciding to Forego Life-Sustaining Treatment* [Washington, D.C.: U.S. Government Printing Office, March, 1983], p. 212, n. 63. Chapter 6 deals with "Seriously Ill Newborns" and offers an excellent survey of ethical issues).

6. F. Raymond Marks, "The Defective Newborn: An Analytic Framework for a Policy Dialog," in Albert R. Jonsen and Michael J. Garland, eds., *Ethics of Newborn Intensive Care* (Berkeley, Calif.: Institute of Governmental Studies, 1976), p. 112.

7. Joseph Fletcher, "The Right to Die," in Paul T. Jersild and Dale A. Johnson, eds., *Moral Issues and Christian Response*, 2nd ed. (New York: Holt, Rinehart and Winston, 1976), p. 398.

8. Sixty-two percent of the total group who believe that children with Down's syndrome "are capable of being useful and bringing love and happiness into the home" would acquiesce in parents' decisions not to allow surgery for atresia (the absence or closure of a body opening). Only 7% who so believe indicate that they would go to court to require surgery (Anthony Shaw, Judson G. Randolph, and Barbara Manard, "Ethical Issues in Pediatric Surgery: A National Survey of Pediatricians and Pediatric Surgeons," *Pediatrics* 60, no. 4 [October 1977]: 596).

9. Michael L. Budde, "There Should Never Be Another Baby Doe," *Washington Post,* 2 April 1983, A 13.

10. Norman Fost, "Counseling Families Who Have a Child with a Severe Congenital Anomaly," *Pediatrics* 67, no. 3 (March 1981): 321.

11. Stanley Hauerwas, *Truthfulness and Tragedy* (Notre Dame: University of Notre Dame Press, 1977), p. 167.

12. Raymond S. Duff, "Counseling Families and Deciding Care of Severely Defective Children: A Way of Coping with 'Medical Vietnam,' " *Pediatrics* 67, no. 3 (March 1981): 319.

13. George J. Annas, "Denying the Rights of the Retarded: The Phillip Becker Case," *Hastings Center Report* 9, no. 6 (December 1979): 18-20. In late September 1983 Phillip received his operation at the insistence of a couple who became his court-appointed (U.S. Supreme Court) legal guardians after having cared for the child for years while he was institutionalized. The operation seems to have been a success.

14. Such a view of ministry is offered by John C. Fletcher, *Coping with Genetic Disease* (San Francisco: Harper & Row, Publishers, 1982), Chap. 2.

15. Said by the parents of Brian West ("Parents Regain Custody of Down's Baby," *Washington Post,* 1 December 1982, A 2).

16. Dr. David McClone; quoted in *Deciding to Forego Life-Sustaining Treatment,* p. 229.

17. Paul Ramsey, *Ethics at the Edges of Life* (New Haven, Conn.: Yale University Press, 1978), p. 215.

18. "Brian West's Short, Tragic Life Is Ended," *Washington Post,* 23 December 1982, A 5.